T0367169

Under the Knife

SAMANTHA KWAN AND
JENNIFER GRAVES

Under the Knife

*Cosmetic Surgery, Boundary Work, and
the Pursuit of the Natural Fake*

TEMPLE UNIVERSITY PRESS
Philadelphia • *Rome* • *Tokyo*

TEMPLE UNIVERSITY PRESS
Philadelphia, Pennsylvania 19122
tupress.temple.edu

Library of Congress Cataloging-in-Publication Data

Names: Kwan, Samantha, author. | Graves, Jennifer, 1983– author.
Title: Under the knife : cosmetic surgery, boundary work, and the pursuit of the
 natural fake / Samantha Kwan and Jennifer Graves.
Description: Philadelphia : Temple University Press, 2020. | Includes bibliographi-
 cal references and index. | Summary: "This book uses interviews with women
 undergoing elective cosmetic surgery to explore the way they make sense of
 their body project in light of dominant cultural discourses, including women's
 agency over their bodies and the undesirability of unnatural aesthetics"—
 Provided by publisher.
Identifiers: LCCN 2019042670 (print) | LCCN 2019042671 (ebook) |
 ISBN 9781439919323 (cloth) | ISBN 9781439919330 (paperback) |
 ISBN 9781439919347 (pdf)
Subjects: LCSH: Body image in women—United States. | Surgery, Plastic—Social
 aspects—United States. | Surgery, Elective—Social aspects—United States. |
 Feminine beauty (Aesthetics)—United States. | Human body—Social aspects—
 United States. | Self perception in women—United States.
Classification: LCC BF697.5.B63 K83 2020 (print) | LCC BF697.5.B63 (ebook) |
 DDC 306.4/613—dc23
LC record available at https://lccn.loc.gov/2019042670
LC ebook record available at https://lccn.loc.gov/2019042671

♾ The paper used in this publication meets the requirements of the American
National Standard for Information Sciences—Permanence of Paper for Printed
Library Materials, ANSI Z39.48-1992

Printed in the United States of America

9 8 7 6 5 4 3 2 1

For Thali, our clock, our tornado, our joy

—SK

For Brenda, my mother, for her unwavering love and support through every battle I've fought

—JG

Contents

Acknowledgments

*U*nder the Knife would not have been possible without our interview participants. We thank them for their time and for sharing their stories with candor. We also thank Ryan Mulligan for his support of our project and his thoughtful editorship, Mary Ann Short for her careful copyediting, and several anonymous reviewers for their insightful comments. We are indebted to Camille Nelson for reference and index preparation, Fanni Farago and Sara Rehman for research assistance, and Wenli Gao for librarian support services. Finally, we extend our appreciation to Scott V. Savage for his patience and support.

Under the Knife

1

The Cosmetic Surgery Paradox

For her fortieth birthday, Marianne,[1] a successful banker in Houston, treated herself to a $15,000 gift. Although she considered herself skinny at 5'3" and 110 pounds, she had, to use her word, "saddlebags." Regardless of how much tennis she played or how often she worked out, she could not get rid of them. Liposuction, she hoped, would do the trick. And since she was going under the knife, she decided she might as well get her breasts done. Marianne had a clear vision of what she wanted out of cosmetic surgery. With liposuction, she desired a more "curvy," "symmetrical," and "proportioned figure." With the breast augmentation, she told us, "I never wanted to look like tits on a stick. . . . I wanted very natural-looking [breasts]." She joked about scoring 100 percent every time she took the "Fake or Real?" quiz—an internet quiz that presents images of women's body parts and then asks viewers to determine if that part has undergone cosmetic surgery. She continued, "It was very important that mine did not look fake."

Marianne is not unique in prioritizing a "natural" outcome. In our interviews with forty-six women who had cosmetic surgery, including Marianne, a concern for natural results emerged as a pervasive theme. *Under the Knife* examines this theme in light of a cultural paradox. On the one hand, a beauty, makeover, and self-improvement culture encourages women to turn to resources within their means—including cosmetic surgery—to improve their appearance. On the other hand, despite increases in the number of some cosmetic surgical procedures among women, cosmetic surgery can still come with stigma. Women who have cosmetic surgery thus face an inherent contradiction—a double bind. Given cultural beauty and self-improvement logics, they attempt to improve their bodies. Yet they potentially face social condemnation for, among other things, being fake or unnatural. So while women are encouraged to take advantage of surgical innovations, there are also social forces that discourage them from doing so. Faced with this contradiction, how do women who have cosmetic surgery resolve this paradox? How do they make sense of and negotiate their "unnatural" surgically altered body?

Body Projects in a Makeover Culture

The pop music icon Madonna purportedly once said, "No matter who you are, no matter what you did, no matter where you've come from, you can always change, become a better version of yourself."[2] These words capture a telling Zeitgeist for women today. There is a cultural imperative for women in America to better themselves. Whether self-help books or reality television programs, a common message emanates from them: Women can improve in all facets of their lives. Whether coordinating the clothes they wear more fashionably or finding their authentic, unique, stable, or true self,[3] they can, as Madonna put it, become a better version of themselves. This is, at least in part, because we live in a makeover culture that rewards people for the work they put into the process of transformation.[4] It is also a culture that exhibits contradictions. For example, despite supposedly being empowered through the process of transformation, one must surrender to experts and authority figures (such as medical doctors and beauty professionals). Additionally, while one wants to be unique, transformation results in looking remarkably like everyone else. This means adopting the appearance of conventional femininity—middle-class, white, ethnically anonymous, and heterosexual.[5]

Because physical attractiveness is inseparable from cultural notions of femininity,[6] for women this self-improvement mandate often centers on appearance. In America, despite subcultural and countercultural ideals, women experience pressure to conform to hegemonic beauty ideals—that is, aesthetic forms exalted as the go-to cultural standards at a given time and place. So at the same time that researchers have documented, for example, black beauty norms and appearance norms among lesbians,[7] there is nevertheless an aesthetic ideal pervasive in fashion magazines and blockbuster Hollywood films.[8] Embodied by A-list actresses such as Anna Kendrick, Jennifer Lawrence, and Emma Watson, it spares no body part from rigid expectations. It demands youthfulness; slenderness; symmetry; coiffed hair; taut, depilated, fair, and unblemished skin; and more.[9] Natural embodiment of this ideal is indisputably a statistical anomaly. One study estimates that the probability of having a body shape similar to real-life Barbie is less than one in one hundred thousand.[10] Everyone knows that most women do not have supermodel Gisele Bündchen's or singer Beyoncé's body! Although embodying these standards is equivalent to winning a genetic lottery of sorts, women still attempt to embody these ideals, in part because there are social expectations that they do so.

Research shows a "beauty bias," in that women who meet these aesthetic demands are often rewarded psychologically, socially, and economically in the form of improved self-esteem, increased dating and marriage opportunities, and higher earnings.[11] Meanwhile, as research on women of size confirms, those who do not meet these aesthetic demands are frequently subject to criticism and even discrimination.[12] People who body shame others often feel justified in their admonishments because makeover projects are not only about the transformation of physical appearance. They are, to borrow the term from social theorist Chris Shilling, *body projects*—"a *project* which should be worked at and accomplished as part of an *individual's* self-identity."[13] These projects involve a process of becoming that is tied to an individual's sense of self. They are self-improvement projects that reflect personal expression—who one is and wants to be.[14] The body that fails to meet beauty standards is purportedly representative of some moral deficiency—a lack of desire, effort, will, or discipline.[15] Subsequently, these "failures" are supposedly deserving of social derision.

In this demanding cultural context, it is not surprising that women feel inordinate pressure to improve their physical appearance. Cosmetic surgery is one of many tools at their disposal.

Cosmetic Surgery in the United States

Cosmetic surgery in the United States is a multibillion-dollar industry, and the latest data indicate that in 2017, Americans spent more than $16.7 billion on cosmetic procedures.[16] The American Society of Plastic Surgeons (ASPS) reports annual statistics by procedures and not people.[17] By ASPS calculations, women in the United States underwent about 92 percent of all cosmetic procedures in 2017, with about 1.4 million procedures involving surgery. (As a reference point, there are about 124 million adult women in the United States.[18]) The most common procedures for women are breast augmentation (augmentation mammoplasty), liposuction, eyelid surgery (blepharoplasty), nose reshaping (rhinoplasty), and tummy tuck (abdominoplasty). Over the last two decades, rates of two of these procedures dramatically increased. Specifically, in 2017, surgeons reported performing 300,378 breast augmentations and 124,869 tummy tucks on women, increases of 41 percent and 107 percent, respectively, since 2000. Table 1.1 presents these data, along with the average surgeon fee associated with each of these procedures.

Cosmetic surgery patients are mostly between the ages of forty and fifty-four.[19] The limited data on socioeconomic status show that about 60 percent of patients have annual household incomes less than $63,000, suggesting that cosmetic surgery is not just a luxury item for the wealthy.[20] ASPS data on demographics reveal that the majority of patients are white. This is the case for women undergoing all major procedures. Table 1.2 contains a breakdown of cosmetic surgical procedures by major racial and ethnic groups in the United States. By and large, white women are the primary consumers of cosmetic surgery. This may be because class is de facto correlated with race and ethnicity in the United States[21] or because researchers have documented more flexible conceptions of beauty among some racial and ethnic minority groups.[22]

TABLE 1.1. MOST COMMON COSMETIC SURGICAL PROCEDURES FOR
WOMEN IN THE UNITED STATES (2017)

Procedure	Number of procedures	Percent change (from 2000 to 2017)	Surgeon fee (national average)*
Breast augmentation	300,378	41	$3,718
Liposuction	218,174	−28	$3,374
Eyelid surgery	177,290	−34	$3,026
Nose reshaping	166,531	−30	$5,125
Tummy tuck	124,869	107	$5,992

Source: ASPS 2018.
* Excludes anesthesia, facility fees, and other related expenses. These averages do not capture how fees can vary considerably by geographic region.

TABLE 1.2. RACIAL AND ETHNIC BREAKDOWN OF COSMETIC
SURGICAL PROCEDURES IN THE UNITED STATES (2017)

Procedure	Caucasian (%)	Hispanic (%)	African American (%)	Asian/ Pacific Islander (%)	Other (%)
Breast augmentation	76	11	6	5	2
Rhinoplasty	75	10	6	4	5
Blepharoplasty	83	7	3	6	2
Liposuction	77	10	8	4	1
Abdominoplasty	70	12	11	5	2

Source: ASPS 2018.
Note: Racial and ethnic labels are those of the American Society of Plastic Surgeons (ASPS 2018).
Blepharoplasty numbers do not add up to 100 percent likely because of rounding error.

Medicalization, Normalization, and a New Aesthetic?

A driving force behind the growth of these procedures, particularly breast augmentation, is the medicalization of women's bodies. Scholars have written at length about the gendered nature of medicalization, arguing that women's bodies and everyday experiences are increasingly subject to medical surveillance.[23] According to the distinguished Brandeis University medical sociologist Peter Conrad, "*Medicalization* describes a process by which nonmedical problems become defined and treated as medical problems, usually in terms of illnesses or disorders."[24] With the medicalization of appearance, people who are unhappy with their looks and who suffer poor body image can use medicine to "correct" and "treat" aesthetic "problems" and "abnormalities."[25] They can turn to medical experts and technologies to "fix" their bodies.[26] Certainly, a long list of medical advances is now available to combat an array of beauty-related problems. We can have our hair transplanted, skin injected with fillers, and discolored skin tempered by laser treatments. We can freeze our fat cells, excise fat and skin, and manipulate the shape and size of our breasts and buttocks. A number of the aesthetic challenges people use medicine to combat are associated with aging.[27] Thinning hair, liver spots, and wrinkles are all a mainstay of growing old. Yet in a makeover and beauty culture, we view these things as unattractive and therefore problematic. Rather than embracing aging, cultural conventions say we should fight its signs, especially given that we have the medical know-how to do so. A profitable medical market driven by private demand provides an endless array of medical services for those who are willing and able to pay.

Medicalization legitimizes cosmetic surgery as an appropriate response to beauty concerns. Surgeons function like psychoanalysts by relieving psychological suffering and improving self-esteem—only, the former work via alterations of the physical body instead of alterations of the mind.[28] With the medicalization of appearance and body image, cosmetic surgery becomes a reasonable solution to body dissatisfaction. Thus, when women define what they perceive to be an aesthetic flaw as a medical problem, they seek a cure, and they are able to feel legitimated in their decision to turn to a surgeon. Of course, whether women's body image can be "fixed" with cosmetic surgery is a different matter, and it is unclear if cosmetic surgery in fact results in improved social-psychological outcomes.[29] In their review of extant research, the psychology professors Charlotte Markey and Patrick Markey conclude, "Cosmetic surgery has the potential to improve women's satisfaction with particular body parts, but it is less likely to improve their overall appearance evaluation and body image."[30]

Within a medicalization paradigm, as the Dutch medical anthropologist Alexander Edmonds observes, one can think of cosmetic surgery as a self-care health practice despite its elective nature. Beauty effectively becomes an "integral dimension of health," and the risks of elective procedures are minimized as they "become absorbed into the medical management of female health."[31] Within this paradigm, one can even argue that elective cosmetic surgery ought to be subsidized, as it is at the Ivo Pitanguy Institute in Rio de Janeiro. Named after the Brazilian plastic surgeon known for saying, "The poor have the right to be beautiful too," the institute—a charity and teaching hospital—provides patients with heavily subsidized or free cosmetic surgery.[32] Similarly, the cosmetic surgery procedures examined by the sociologist Kathy Davis in her groundbreaking research in the Netherlands were covered by Dutch national health insurance.[33]

Whether publicly subsidized or not, with "aesthetic medicine," beauty and health become entangled.[34] Yet this is precisely the concern expressed by critics. Historical and contemporary social intolerance of "abnormal" appearance means that next to everyone falls outside aesthetic norms and *needs* medicine's help to correct physical appearance.[35] As a society, we no longer tolerate aesthetic diversity. Instead, as the renowned University of Toronto philosophy professor Kathryn Pauly Morgan argues in her influential ruminations on cosmetic surgery, we pathologize minor deviations from beauty ideals and label "problem areas" as "ugly," describing them as "deformities" in need of medical correction.[36] Moreover, cosmetic surgery can result in the medicalization of racial features. For example, Eugenia Kaw's anthropological research involving interviews with physicians and patients shows how Asian American women internalize a racial and gendered ideology constructed by Western media.[37] This ideology, which surgeons promote to increase demand, constructs these women's natural physical features as undesirable (because it culturally signifies dullness and passivity) and in need of medical correction through, say, eyelid or nose bridge restructuring. Research also shows that medicalization is gendered insofar as surgeons see surgery as "normal" and "natural" for women but not for men.[38] Again, the message remains: The beauty mandate is almost exclusively a woman's mandate.

Industry growth has led some scholars to argue that cosmetic surgery has been normalized or domesticated.[39] They point out that, over the last three decades, there has been a "mainstreaming of cosmetic surgery techniques and procedures in Westernized societies," and today "*everybody* knows about cosmetic surgery."[40] This normalization is evident in the growing number of procedures, the ubiquity of surgically altered celebrities, and the emergence and growth of cosmetic-surgery-focused reality television programs since the early 2000s.[41] The internet is now abuzz with gossip about which celebrity had this nipped and that tucked. Notably, this discussion is often rife with judgment and negative assumptions about both motive and character. Morgan even speculates that women who contemplate *not* having surgery will be subject to stigma,[42] while other scholars maintain that there may be a new coveted aesthetic of artificiality, particularly with breast enhancement, that allows women to conspicuously display upward mobility.[43] She ventures that the pervasiveness of aesthetic technologies will one day mean that the "naturally 'given'" will increasingly come to be viewed as "technologically 'primitive'" and that "ordinary" will eventually be perceived as "ugly."[44]

Stigma and Cosmetic Surgery

Despite some procedures becoming more common, medicalization, the claim of a new cosmetic surgery aesthetic, and cosmetic surgery's pervasiveness in everyday discourses, a veil of stigma still surrounds the cosmetic surgery industry and its patients. Stigma, as the sociologist Erving Goffman has long described it, is an attribute that is discrediting.[45] The stigma of cosmetic surgery has historical roots. At the turn of the twentieth century, those who were conducting invasive medical procedures that would today be labeled cosmetic surgery had quite a spotty reputation. Reputable surgeons accused these practitioners of placing healthy patients at risk and performing medical interventions that contradicted "the traditional American injunction against vanity," as well as the Hippocratic oath to do no harm. The historian Elizabeth Haiken documents that "'beauty surgery' was the province of quacks and charlatans."[46] In the industry's initial stages of development, cosmetic surgery earned the unfortunate reputation of being "dirty work." Practitioners and clients alike were perceived as socially deviant.[47]

Over time, efforts to increase the profession's legitimacy have been somewhat successful, with professional organizations playing a pivotal role in this transformation.[48] For example, the formation of the American Association of Plastic Surgeons in 1921 helped define boundaries of acceptable practice, set standards, and regulate practitioners.[49] These organizations eventually collected data on their clientele and began marketing extensively to their new consumer base.[50] New social norms that emphasized beauty and individuality, along with the medicalization of appearance, further added to the industry's legitimacy.[51] Today, the industry has mostly moved out of the "domain of the sleazy, the suspicious, the secretively deviant, or the pathologically narcissistic."[52]

Even with this cleaner reputation, the cosmetic surgery profession still experiences reputational struggles. For example, research in the United States and abroad finds that the public, along with other medical professionals, grossly underestimates the scope of this specialty.[53] Specifically, individuals do not typically identify cosmetic surgeons as having broad and extensive technical skills but rather associate them exclusively with procedures used to enhance aesthetic appearance. Narrow media depictions of the profession, such as FX's *Nip/Tuck*, have done little to enhance the reputation of cosmetic surgeons. This TV drama graphically depicted surgeries while following the lives of two cosmetic surgeons, including their sexual exploits, sometimes even with patients. After *Nip/Tuck*'s debut, professional organizations representing board-certified surgeons posted press releases on their websites condemning the show.[54] These efforts are worthwhile, as research finds that such shows do in fact negatively affect the public's perception of the profession.[55] Indeed, some cosmetic surgeons recognize that their specialty requires defending. One Seattle-based surgeon goes as far as to include on his surgery center's website a blurb titled "Clearing Up Stereotypes about Plastic Surgeons." In it, he insists that it is "not about fancy cars and dating beautiful woman [sic] . . . [or] the money." Rather, it is about "the positive impact that they can make on their patients' lives."[56]

Stigma surrounds patients, too. Scholars document that cosmetic surgery has been historically associated with a list of undesirable characteristics including immorality, narcissism, and psychological maladjustment.[57] Contemporary studies show that the public still holds negative views of cosmetic surgery patients, perceiving them as psychologically maladjusted and associating them with low self-esteem, materialism, self-consciousness, perfectionism, and the unnatural.[58] One opinion piece by several plastic surgeons published in *Plastic and Reconstructive Surgery* opens with "There is, without a question, a stigma in American culture attached to cosmetic surgery and a hidden condescension toward patients undergoing these procedures." The authors criticize mass media for perpetuating this stigma, speculating that "the stigma in American culture has to do with disrupting antiquated, classicist ideals that beauty is something with which one is born."[59] Until society is rid of the assumption that people are only born beautiful, they maintain, beauty bought will continue to be tainted. These surgeons question why beauty purchased or facilitated by surgery is devalued or loses its luster. Their words, no doubt, are a defense of the medicalization of beauty.

A qualitative study by psychologists in England and Australia sheds light on cosmetic surgery stigma by revealing how public indictment of breast implants operates on two levels.[60] First, negative evaluations of surgically enhanced breasts center on their aesthetic unnaturalness and the visibility of augmentation. These researchers observed that people rebuke the results of breast enhancement surgery for looking like "rockhard fake gazongas," having a "plastic blow up doll look," and appearing like "robot tits."[61] Yet this aesthetic inferiority, they argue, is just a springboard for a second indictment of "the personalities of women who have breast augmentation . . . [who are construed] as deceptive or deviant."[62] Supposedly, breast implants reveal something about a woman who has them. For example, cosmetic surgery implies that she is a "superficial bimbo," "trying too hard," has "confidence issues," or suffers from "low self-esteem."[63]

A 2016 report by the Pew Research Center, a nonpartisan Washington, DC, think tank, further confirms public disapproval of cosmetic surgery. The report maintains that "public opinion [is] mostly negative on [the] use of cosmetic procedures today."[64] Accompanying this claim, the center reports that almost two-thirds of those surveyed say that individuals are too quick to undergo cosmetic procedures and only 16 percent say these procedures have more benefits than downsides.[65]

It is important to point out that cosmetic surgery in the United States remains uncommon. Yes, more people are turning to it. Everybody seems to know about it. Coverage of it in mainstream media is rampant. Yet in their lifetimes most Americans will not undergo cosmetic surgery. In reality, only 4 percent of adult Americans have ever had elective cosmetic surgery.[66] It is statistically rare. And because the main consumers are white women, it is even rarer among men and people of color.[67] People who undergo cosmetic surgery, even white women, are not the statistical norm. In fact, they constitute a minority.

So while a makeover culture encourages women to pursue body projects to better themselves, women who turn to cosmetic surgery potentially encounter a conundrum. They attempt to improve their bodies to align with cultural standards but may face social stigma for, among other things, being fake or unnatural. *Under the Knife* explores how women resolve this paradox, especially within the context of ongoing feminist debates about cosmetic surgery.

Feminist Perspectives

Choice and Empowerment

Some popular depictions and discussions of cosmetic surgery take a more laudatory approach.[68] They do this by positively framing cosmetic surgery as "scientific progress," "innovation," and a tool that provides a "cure for suffering and a route to empowerment."[69] For example, cosmetic-surgery-focused reality television programs depict women as autonomous self-determining individuals who elect surgery.[70] As rational actors, women choose cosmetic surgery to better themselves.

Such framing is emblematic of postfeminist rhetoric. Although multifaceted, postfeminism suggests an end to feminism as a movement on the premise that women no longer need it.[71] Ostensibly, this is because the postfeminist woman is an empowered and active (including sexually active) subject in both her public and her private life.[72] Epitomized by Kim Kardashian, she chooses her destiny and, if she fancies, even to be objectified.[73] This line of thinking maintains that women can use beauty practices, including cosmetic surgery, to embody sexiness and to gain erotic capital for the sake of advancement.[74] Choice—whether it is the right to choose sexual encounters, make health decisions, or elect cosmetic surgery—is a cherished principle at the heart of neoliberal consumerist and postfeminist culture.[75]

Postfeminist discourses are part of a makeover culture that emphasizes the achieved self, mostly in the pursuit of beauty and body perfection.[76] Popular cultural references depict the postfeminist woman as educated and successful in the workplace. Yet she is preoccupied with adornment.[77] Her economic successes enable her to adorn herself with Jimmy Choo heels, Hermès scarves, and Burberry handbags. She is embodied by *Sex and the City*'s Carrie.[78] At the core of postfeminism is thus consumerism and particularly consumption in the name of beauty and fashion.[79] Cosmetic surgery is merely one of many tools on the consumer beauty market a woman can purchase to achieve her desired self. In fact, the communication scholars Sarah Banet-Weiser and Laura Portwood-Stacer view the increasing use of cosmetic surgery as *the* quintessential expression of postfeminism. This is because cosmetic surgery legitimizes idealized feminine beauty and is the quintessential articulation of individual transformation and empowerment. They observe that makeover TV shows stress the "pleasure of transforming the self" and "becoming a better 'you' by making better purchases and adopting better lifestyle habits."[80]

The first major theoretical lens on cosmetic surgery therefore frames cosmetic surgery as a scientific innovation that *empowers* women. Rational women elect surgery to open up opportunities and gain various forms of capital.[81] They are not victims of fashion magazines and Hollywood productions. Rather, they are, according to the sociologist Debra Gimlin, "savvy cultural negotiators."[82] They turn to beauty as a means to achieve psychological, social, and material rewards. Women use beauty, for example, to renegotiate their relationship with their bodies and to construct a certain sense of self. The work by one sociologist who has studied cosmetic surgery extensively confirms this. Kathy Davis finds that cosmetic surgery enables women to take control of their lives, to feel normal, and to obtain a body to which they feel entitled.[83]

Conformity and Oppression

In contrast, some scholars point out that this choice and empowerment rhetoric obscures power dynamics.[84] In reality, what are supposedly freely made choices are constrained. Choices are never made in a vacuum but are made within a social context. A beauty hierarchy, created and reinforced through media discourses, as well as everyday talk, deems some bodies physically attractive and labels others as unattractive. A self-improvement makeover culture and a beauty hierarchy that rewards conformity to hegemonic ideals create compelling social forces. Women feel pressure to conform to beauty ideals, especially in the absence of strong alternative beauty ideals. In this context, women may feel that there is only one choice—to conform.[85] In the end, choice looks a lot like conformity and acquiescence.[86] From this perspective, cosmetic surgery is not empowering but a form of oppression and discipline to gendered and racialized beauty ideals.[87] This oppression works in insidious ways—not through overt coercion but through self-surveillance.[88] Women voluntarily comply, participating willingly in their own subjugation.

Critics of the choice and empowerment lens further contend that while cosmetic surgery may result in individual empowerment, these are personal-level gains. These gains do little to challenge social and cultural ideologies.[89] One woman's use of cosmetic surgery may help improve her life circumstances by, say, upping her chances of finding a romantic partner or advancing in the workplace. However, this personal choice fails to challenge sexist ideologies that equate women's bodies with their identities or reward women's bodies over their intellects.[90] Cosmetic surgery also means the ongoing reification of hegemonic beauty ideals.[91] As more women try to embody the ideal, the more tangible and visible it becomes. From this perspective, although women have the free will to opt out of cosmetic surgery, the practice is not empowering to women as a collective.[92] It results in the reproduction, not the transformation, of an oppressive beauty culture.[93]

Victimization is at the heart of this second lens. This lens stresses how beauty ideals support patriarchal and capitalist institutions,[94] emphasizing that women who undergo cosmetic surgery have false consciousness.[95] They are supposedly complicit in and oblivious to their own oppression. They are not empowered agents but oppressed victims who embody beauty ideals for the male gaze.[96] To boot, this lens emphasizes that these ideals are not only unrealistic and unattainable; they can cause physical, psychological, and emotional damage.[97] They also reinforce racism, ageism, ableism, and classism, because the norms themselves presuppose a white, youthful, and able body.[98] Cosmetic surgery can erase racial and ethnic identifiers.[99] And its embodiment requires financial and time investments—a luxury that favors the socioeconomically privileged. Low-income minority women who are not able to invest in the ideal lose out on economic mobility and other social benefits.[100]

While the empowerment-oppression debate informs contemporary research on cosmetic surgery, some scholars argue for the decentering of the subject. For example, the body scholar Victoria Pitts-Taylor proposes moving past the question of "is she victimized, or empowered?"[101] This is because "the subjectivity of the cosmetic surgery patient is not fixed but rather fluid" and the "personal is implicated in the larger social relations of cosmetic surgery."[102] Instead, she suggests that researchers examine *how* these social relations—including medical, popular culture, and interpersonal discourses about cosmetic surgery—continuously shape the way the self is constituted.[103]

Making Sense of and Negotiating an "Unnatural" Body

It is in consideration of these competing lenses and the larger social relations that dynamically shape the self that we aim to understand women's meaning making about their bodies. The pages that follow reveal how women negotiate their "unnatural"—but, they hope, natural looking—surgically altered bodies. Specifically, *Under the Knife* focuses on several interrelated social psychological processes. As we saw in Marianne's chapter-opening preoperative sentiments, participants desire the "natural fake"—a discreet alteration of the body that appears as if it were achieved without surgical intervention. This natural fake allows them to pass as surgically unaltered. Participants also negotiate their postoperative bodies via their definitions of *natural* and the *natural body*. Moreover, they create boundaries between themselves and discredited others who undergo surgery. Finally, when they encounter problems and surgery does not deliver the natural fake, they turn to various management strategies. Ultimately, these strategies—of passing, redefining, boundary work, and physical and psychological management—are essential for identity management and allow participants to preserve a distinctly gendered, authentic, and moral self.

Interviews with Women Who Go Under the Knife

Our findings are based on in-depth interviews with forty-six women who underwent cosmetic surgery. Using the definitions provided by the American Board of Cosmetic Surgery, we recruited participants who were "focused on enhancing appearance" rather than those "repairing defects to reconstruct a normal function and appearance."[104] Study participants must have been, to some degree, motivated to enhance their aesthetic appearance, even if surgery served some functional or health benefit (such as greater mobility or less chaffing). Procedures also had to involve surgery, thereby excluding nonsurgical procedures such as Botox (botulinum toxin) injections, microdermabrasion, and laser hair removal.[105]

Participants' surgeries were elective in that the procedures they underwent were not immediately lifesaving. Cosmetic surgery is never needed to save someone's life. However, the concept of elective surgery itself involves contested boundaries, as the sociologist Heather Laine Talley's work illustrates. Talley argues that the distinction between "optimization and repair, cosmetic and reconstruction, seems to be eroding."[106] Her research on facial work shows how aesthetic surgery, such as face transplant surgery, can be interpreted as lifesaving work. This is because appearance difference can amount to a form of social death—a cessation of social viability—and facial surgery is considered humanizing in light of the detrimental social consequences of facial disfigurement.[107] Thus, in Chapter 4 we elucidate how participants often define their surgeries as necessary and complicate the notion that cosmetic surgery is elective.

We recruited participants through a wide variety of techniques, including advertisements on cosmetic surgery message boards, at local fitness and athletics establishments, and in surgeon's offices.[108] Yet it was often through word of mouth that participants found out about the study. While we did not intend to interview only women and we doubled efforts to find men by reaching out to surgeons known to cater to men, our final sample consisted entirely of women, reflecting the reality that women undergo the vast majority of all cosmetic surgery procedures in the United States.

We conducted interviews in California and Texas between summer 2014 and fall 2015. We each conducted about half the interviews, which took one to two and a half hours each.[109] Our questions covered a broad range of topics related to participants' surgery experiences and views—from the decision-making processes to adjusting to life after surgery. We digitally recorded all interviews, which were conducted in either an office or a location of the participant's choosing (such as a coffee shop).

We transcribed about a dozen recordings before turning to a professional transcription service that provided verbatim transcripts. We found the transcripts quite accurate, as interviews did not involve extensive medical terminology and were akin to a casual yet directed conversation. We coded these transcripts using the software program Atlas.ti. Our inductive approach, informed by grounded theory, focused on exploring themes and fleshing out social processes.[110] Because we adapted our interview guide to emergent theoretical developments, not all questions were posed to all participants. Consequently, and because our goal is not statistical representation, we generally do not report numbers, avoiding the misleading implication that these numbers might reflect some statistical pattern in a larger population. Our careful, thorough, and systematic treatment of data, along with our familiarity with social scientific scholarship on the body, make us confident our data, findings, and interpretations reflect empirical processes at work in the social world. We also believe our positionality increased the validity of our data and analysis more than it compromised it.[111] We challenge quantitative researchers to test formal hypotheses derived from our findings and encourage other qualitative researchers to further flesh out our theoretical claims.

Who Are Our Participants?

Of the forty-six women we interviewed, ten resided in California and the rest in Texas. Their ages ranged from twenty to sixty-eight, with an average age of thirty-nine. Similar to national patient demographics, twenty-eight (or 61 percent) identified as white, ten (or 22 percent) as Hispanic, four (or 9 percent) as African American, three (or 7 percent) as East Asian or Pacific Islander, and one (or 2 percent) as Middle Eastern.[112] Thus, eighteen women (or 39 percent) in our sample identified as women of color. While this small number of women of color does not permit elaborate claims about the role race or ethnicity has on cosmetic surgery, we nevertheless point out racialized themes and social processes when the evidence presents itself. In addition to racial and ethnic diversity, our sample exhibits socioeconomic diversity. Twenty-two (or 48 percent) had some college education or were currently working toward a college degree, while another seventeen (or 37 percent) had completed a baccalaureate degree. Five (or 11 percent) had a master's or professional degree, while the remaining two (or 4 percent) had a high school degree or its equivalent. Participants had a range of occupations. Some were administrative assistants, sales representatives, and managers (at banks, restaurants, and medical offices). Others worked in professional careers such as teaching, medicine, dentistry, and interior design. Personal annual income data reflect the diversity in participants' education and occupation. Eight (or 17 percent) earned less than $19,999. Ten (or 22 percent) earned between $20,000 and $39,999, eight (or 17 percent) earned between $40,000 and $59,000, ten (or 22 percent) earned between $60,000 and $79,999, four (or 9 percent) earned between $80,000 and $99,999, and the remaining five (or 11 percent) earned more than $100,000.[113] Notably, all five women with personal annual incomes greater than $100,000 identified as white.

About a quarter of the women were married at the time of their interviews. Two participants were engaged. Just over a third were either single or widowed at the time of their interviews. Sixteen (or 37 percent) had divorced at some time in their lives. Twenty-two (or 48 percent) did not have children, while ten (or 22 percent) had one. The remaining fourteen (or 30 percent) had two or more children. The majority (forty-three, or 94 percent) identified as heterosexual, while the rest identified as bisexual. There is a cisgender bias in our sample, as no participant revealed a lack of correspondence between her gender identity and birth sex.

The age when participants had surgery varied. In an attempt to understand both short- and long-term processes, we placed no study restrictions on when participants underwent surgery. For example, we interviewed Darla, age twenty-seven, two months after she had rhinoplasty. In contrast, we interviewed Jessica, age sixty-eight, who had had her first surgery—breast augmentation—forty-three years earlier, in 1972.

The type and number of procedures participants had also varied. Similar to national trends, the most common surgery among participants was breast augmentation (twenty-six women, or 57 percent).[114] This was followed by liposuction and rhinoplasty (both were done by eleven women, or 24 percent) and abdominoplasty (nine women, or 20 percent). Four women (9 percent) had some form of a face-lift.[115] Participants also had the following procedures alone or in combination with another cosmetic procedure: breast reduction (two women), eyelid surgery (one woman), jaw surgery (one woman), otoplasty (ear surgery) (one woman), and some form of a body lift or tuck (five women).[116] In the Appendix, we present a table that includes each participant's pseudonym, key demographics, and the procedures she underwent.

The most common procedure for the women of color in our sample was breast augmentation, which eight of them had. This was followed by abdominoplasty (five), rhinoplasty (four), and liposuction (three). The most common procedure for the white women in our sample was also breast surgery, which eighteen had. This was followed by liposuction (eight), rhinoplasty (seven), abdominoplasty (four), and face-lift (four). Table 1.3 presents a breakdown of procedures by racial and ethnic category.

It is noteworthy that the surgeries participants underwent would not be considered racialized procedures. The sociologist Margaret Hunter describes "racial capital" as a resource drawn from the body related to skin tone, facial features, and body shape within the context

TABLE 1.3. NUMBER OF PARTICIPANTS' PROCEDURES BY RACIAL AND ETHNIC CATEGORY

	Breast augmenta-tion	Rhino-plasty	Lipo-suction	Abdomino-plasty	Face-lift
Women of color (n = 18)	8	4	3	5	0
White women (n = 28)	18	7	8	4	4

of existing racial hierarchies.[117] The cosmetic industry sells this capital, she argues, in the form of "Anglo noses, Anglo eyes" while simultaneously maintaining that patients are preserving their racial or ethnic identity.[118] For some patients, then, cosmetic surgery, such as blepharoplasty (eyelid surgery), *can* have deeper meanings about race and ethnicity. For example, double-eyelid surgery for an East Asian woman may be highly racialized, unlike eyelid surgery for a woman of European descent to remove bags around her eyes. Yet this was not the case with our participants. The only participant in our sample who had eyelid surgery, Penelope, a white woman, said she wanted to preserve a more youthful look, stating she did not like the appearance of these bags. Moreover, when participants discussed an array of issues about cosmetic surgery (including motivations and beauty culture in general), none explicitly framed their desire for noses, breasts, or other body parts in terms of their racial or ethnic identity. Instead, they simply wanted more aesthetically pleasing body parts. By and large, our participants viewed surgery through a gendered lens. As Chapter 2 underscores, motivations for cosmetic surgery are predominantly about living up to aesthetic norms of femininity, while racial and ethnic discourses are secondary at best.

At the time of their interview, just over two-thirds of participants (thirty-two, or 70 percent) had had a single unique procedure, meaning that about one-third had two or more procedures, sometimes three or more. For example, when we met Lena at age forty-four she had had rhinoplasty at age eighteen, followed by breast augmentation at twenty-five, and then a second breast augmentation at thirty-six. The self-reported average age of first surgery was approximately twenty-nine.[119]

Nine women (or 20 percent) had several surgeries of the same type. In the majority of these cases, participants were either dissatisfied with the results or encountered physical problems (such as leakage in a breast implant).[120] All but four participants had surgery in the United States. One participant had surgery in the Middle East because a close relative was an experienced and reputable surgeon whom the participant trusted. The other three participants went to Latin America because they felt they were saving a significant amount of money.

Plan of the Book

To understand how women resolve the cosmetic surgery paradox, we first turn to their decision to go under the knife. The decision is a serious one with, as makeover discourses intimate, supposedly life-altering consequences. Chapter 2 is thus the first of four chapters that set the empirical foundation of the book. In this chapter, we examine women's motivations for surgery and the stigma surrounding cosmetic surgery. We document why women pursue cosmetic surgery and their concerns about having chosen a form of body modification that comes with social rebuke. These concerns lead them to desire a very specific surgical outcome—the natural fake.

In Chapter 3, we examine participants' pursuit of this natural fake and their understandings of *natural*. What exactly are natural surgical results, and after surgery do the women consider their bodies natural? Our interviews revealed that participants associate natural surgical results with what is God-given, with what is not artificially altered, and with inconspicuousness, and that they frame natural surgical results as feminine enhancement and restoration. Moreover, their accounts of their postoperative bodies as still "natural" or "natural looking" constitute a form of passing and one strategy participants use to manage the cosmetic surgery paradox.

Chapter 4 focuses on another strategy. Participants justify their altered bodies and their decision to have cosmetic surgery by creating boundaries between good and bad surgery and between good and bad patients. They construct an image of a good patient as a well-adjusted, psychologically balanced woman who uses surgery to achieve normative femininity and to empower herself. In this way, women who have cosmetic surgery turn the table on the paradox by taking a moral high ground. In a self-improvement makeover culture, they are merely good female citizens seeking to better themselves. Chapter 4 is therefore an in-depth look at boundary work and how this work enables participants to preserve a moral self that also allows them to stay true to themselves.

Does surgery live up to expectations? If women desire the natural fake, are they pleased with the results? Chapter 5 examines what happens after surgery. While the majority of participants were generally content with their decision to have surgery, there were nevertheless complications and disappointments, including the disappointment that surgery did not deliver the natural fake. Chapter 5 describes some of the psychological and physical strategies participants used to manage these complications and disappointments. It also shines light on the stories of several participants who exhibited a fraught relationship with cosmetic surgery. Their stories illustrate that disappointment with cosmetic surgery can lead to challenges, albeit limited, to the same beauty norms that prompted the initial decision to go under the knife.

Chapter 6 summarizes our main empirical findings within the context of extant research and discusses why all this matters. Ultimately, *Under the Knife* highlights the role of deep-seated yet contradictory gendered meanings about women's bodies. Strategies of passing, redefining, boundary work, and physical and psychological management enable women to preserve an authentic and gendered moral self—a self that, despite the articulation of empowerment rhetoric, comports with traditional notions of femininity and virtue.

Motivations and Concerns

I'm grateful that we have Western medicine and the procedures available to us so that I could feel and look normal.

—HEATHER

They can't judge you for having natural large breasts. But
then when you go and get a boob job, it's different.

—CHARLIZE

C ultural debates and discourses about self-improvement,
beauty, and stigma provide an important backdrop for understanding women's relationship with cosmetic surgery and
their bodies. Yet a thorough understanding requires hearing from
the women themselves. We shift our focus now to participants'
voices. What motivated them to make this decision? And are they
concerned about the social disapproval that might come with such
a decision?

Motivations

Participants did not take lightly the decision to have cosmetic surgery. While a handful contemplated surgery for only a few weeks, the
majority considered it for many years.[1] In fact, almost a fifth of our
participants said they thought about the procedure for more than ten
years. No doubt the decision is fraught with fear and anxiety. These
fears and anxieties concern the stigma of undergoing elective surgery
that is not lifesaving, as well as the usual concerns about undergoing
any surgical procedure. Commonly expressed trepidations include

the fear of needles, physical pain, implant rupture, infection, potential addiction to pain medications, and death.[2]

Participants also wrestled with the cost of surgery. Following national trends, the most common surgical procedure among our participants was breast augmentation. While national averages are about $3,513 for saline implants and $4,014 for silicone gel implants,[3] our participants reported paying between $2,500 and $8,000, with about half electing saline and half electing silicone.[4] About 80 percent paid for their surgeries without institutional financing, sometimes with the help of a family member. Most participants expressed awareness that surgery consumed a large amount of discretionary income. Some described how they "worked hard," "saved," and "scraped together" the money. Grace took on a second job specifically to pay for surgery, while Jasmine funded her surgeries by sacrificing the money her mom was planning to give her as a wedding gift. Sylvia and Taylor purposely had their surgeries abroad to reduce costs. For those who turned to institutional financing, this meant putting all or a portion of the surgery cost on a credit card.[5] In Caitlin's case, it meant financing her breast augmentation through a student loan. Regardless of payment form, participants acknowledged that it was not an insignificant chunk of change to spend on beauty.[6]

So what motivates women to have cosmetic surgery despite the physical and social risks and financial burden? Researchers have documented a slew of reasons, typically framing motivations in light of the empowerment-oppression debate discussed in Chapter 1. On the one hand, they observe that women, as autonomous and active subjects who exercise free will, use surgery as a tool to achieve some end. This end might be social-psychological such as increased self-esteem or body satisfaction. It might be economic and pertain to upward mobility in the workplace. Or it might be social and involve increased opportunities in the marriage marketplace. On the other hand, outside influences, such as social networks, media, and medical discourses, also affect the decision to have cosmetic surgery.[7] Participants indicated that both internal and external factors, but especially the desire to achieve normative femininity and reap its rewards, shaped their decision to have cosmetic surgery.[8]

Achieving Normalcy, Embodying Womanhood

While media images link cosmetic surgery to the glitz and glamour of Hollywood, participants did not turn to cosmetic surgery because they coveted the glamorous life. Rather, similar to extant research reporting that cosmetic surgery patients desire normalcy,[9] they turned to surgery to be "normal," to use their word. For example, at age twenty, Heather had breast augmentation to fix what she considered uneven breasts. Living in Southern California, she also wanted to be "a little fuller" while wearing swimsuits and workout clothes. She approached her mom to talk about her body discontentment, and, to her surprise, her mom disclosed that she had breast implants. A conversation ensued, and Heather's mom eventually encouraged Heather to have surgery and even agreed to pay for it.

Now age thirty-eight and a high school health teacher, Heather reflected on her motives for cosmetic surgery: "I just want[ed] to be normal . . . to feel and look normal," she said. Having even breasts, she believed, would allow her to do everyday things and "not [feel] like a freak." She expressed frustration that before surgery she had to wear padded and "weird bras" and, when working out, loose clothing. Going to the beach held little appeal because it elicited anxiety and led to the menacing question of "Well, um, how am I going to handle this?" Surgery provided "freedom" and allowed her to participate in the mundane. She no longer felt restricted in her clothing choices. She now had the freedom to navigate public spaces, including the gym and the beach, with less anxiety.

The desire for normalcy was a sentiment expressed by other participants. For example, at age twenty-two, Elaina had nose and ear surgery. She did not want to be "the oddball that sticks out: 'Oh yeah, the one with the funny ears.'" Similarly, Barbara's surgery was about "blending in, fitting in." Despite saying that "there is no such thing as normal," she nevertheless maintained that her trunk lift at age fifty-two allowed her to "go out and just be another person in the crowd." Reese, who had breast augmentation at age nineteen, also felt that surgery is not about standing out: "I just wanted to look normal, like most people."

Cosmetic surgery enables women to blend into the crowd and achieve normalcy. Yet closer examination reveals that this achievement is gendered. Specifically, they seek to embody normative femininity.[10] As scholars have documented, cosmetic surgery allows women to reaffirm femininity[11] and "do gender."[12] According to the sociologists Candace West and Don Zimmerman, gender is a routine accomplishment of social doings embedded in everyday interactions. Every day, individuals manipulate their appearance, behavior, demeanor, and speech (among other things) to comport with normative conceptions of femininity and masculinity. West and Zimmerman maintain that because our sex category (gender cues that suggest one is female or male) is omnirelevant, nearly all our daily activities are held accountable to these normative conceptions. We are always doing gender.

A long list of behaviors, comportments, and embodiments is certainly associated with femininity. And where appearance is concerned, there is no shortage of rules about what women's bodies ought to look like.[13] Participants have a clear idea of how they should and want to appear, and while they have no expectation that they will look like a *Vogue* model, they nevertheless believe an adult woman should possess certain physical features, such as fair and unblemished skin, svelteness (but not so thin as to suggest a clinical diagnosis such as anorexia nervosa), ample breasts, and a low waist-to-hip ratio. Simply put, they should look less like a model from a seventeenth-century Rubens painting[14] and more like Kendall Jenner, who by Forbes' accounting was the highest-paid model of 2018.[15]

Reese's description of a mismatch between her psyche and physical body illustrates how cosmetic surgery allows women to achieve normative femininity. At age nineteen she obtained implants to transform her breasts from, in terms of bra sizes, "negative A" to 32DD.[16] She had considered having cosmetic surgery since her preteens but moved forward with it only after her grandmother died and left her some money. When she broached the topic with her mom, Reese, like Heather, was surprised to discover that her mom too had a history of cosmetic surgery. Reese felt that, because her mom had breast surgery and a face-lift, she was empathetic. For this reason, she surmised, her mom agreed to pay for half the surgery cost.

Reese was motivated by the desire to look feminine, telling us that before surgery she did not feel feminine despite being born biologically female. She compared herself to two transgender friends who were transitioning. One underwent sex change surgery and the other was undergoing hormone therapy. The transitioning process, she believed, helped her friends align how they feel on the inside with how they appear on the outside:

> I think, it's like, it would make them more the person they are inside—their body could reflect [it]. So I feel kinda the same. I guess I linked it to that because I did feel more like a guy before. Not that I had a penis or anything. But I just had more of an upper torso of a man, and I knew it would never change.

She described having "innies," "no boobs at all," and a chest cavity that caved inward. So from a young age, she always felt like a "tomboy" and "odd in [her] own body," and she would wear "just guy clothes." Surgery was largely about the embodiment of womanhood. Surgery made her "realize that [she's] a woman," and she "can dress like a woman now." For Reese, surgery helped align how she looks on the outside (i.e., like an endowed woman) with how she wanted to, and believed she was supposed to, feel on the inside (i.e., feminine).

Reese is not alone in this belief. Many participants, especially those who underwent breast surgery, felt they failed to live up to cultural templates of womanhood. When discussing her motivations for breast augmentation, Jessica lamented, "I didn't feel feminine looking. . . . I just didn't feel like a woman." Carla, even after giving birth to three children, "felt like a little girl because [she] didn't have much breasts." Kristen stated, "Honestly, I felt like a twelve-year-old. I felt like a girl. I knew I was twenty-three, but I didn't feel like it." Ashley echoed similar motives for her breast surgery: "I just felt like I wasn't a full woman. I felt like a child . . . like I looked like a boy, . . . underdeveloped. It's like a weirdo, like a freak, really." Meanwhile, Kaylee remarked candidly, "Real women have curves."

Cosmetic surgery not only helps women embody cultural ideals of femininity; it enables them to *feel* feminine. Cultural discourses in the United States construct a physical ideal of women that emphasizes curves, especially large breasts.[17] With breast augmentation, women can align their external appearance with a feminine sense of self. With surgery, they can feel like a woman, a "normal" woman. Importantly, however, participants made clear that it is not about pursuing a hypersexualized ideal—an observation we expand on in Chapter 4. Rather, it is about the embodiment of *ordinary* womanhood. For example, Kristen said, "I wanted to feel like a woman. I don't have to be like va-va-voom. I wasn't going for that. I just wanted a little bit of oomph." Surgery enabled her to possess a physical feature, specifically larger breasts, to signify to others, as well as herself, that she is a woman. Moreover, *looking* like a woman meant she could *feel* like a woman—mature, beautiful, sexy, and desirable. In the words of Ana Marie, who also obtained breast implants, "You cannot be sexy if you don't have boobs." Or as Carla said, "I was cute when I was younger, but I never felt pretty and wanted. . . . I never *felt* sexy. I finally [with breast implants] *felt* sexy."[18]

Cultural Ideals: "We Have This Image Stuck in Our Heads"

The desire to achieve normative femininity points to the pervasiveness of a hegemonic ideal of femininity despite the existence of subcultural ideals. So even when some communities promote, say, acceptance of larger body sizes, there is still a prevalent feminine ideal of thinness venerated by mass media. While there is some debate as to whether this ideal has its roots in evolutionary psychology or cultural institutions,[19] some scholars maintain that media images play a key role.[20] Participants confirmed this. For one, they admitted looking at fashion magazines, especially in their youth, and being regularly exposed to beauty ideals online and on television. Regarding women's breast standards, Kerrie, who had breast augmentation at age twenty-seven, confessed, "I guess it's, growing up, you see all these women on television and magazines, and they're just perky. Even though they're airbrushed and Photoshopped like crazy, but we have this image stuck in our heads. Like this is the way that girls are supposed to be." Like Kerrie, many participants exhibited cultural savvy, recognizing that media images are doctored. Fashion models in magazines are, as they said, "Photoshopped," while Hollywood images are "not real," "unrealistic," and "unattainable." Despite this shrewd understanding that women's beauty ideals are largely media-constructed fictions, these ideals nonetheless shape their vision of what a woman's body should look like. In other words, participants admitted feeling this cultural pressure even though their media savviness suggests that they are not "cultural dopes"[21] who lack agency and blindly follow cultural norms. Jessica's words are telling. In a single breath, she made a direct connection between media images and how she sees herself: "You see all the women in the pictures. I wasn't curvy like a woman."

Some participants, like Claronette, age fifty-nine, were up front about how mass media influenced their decision to have cosmetic surgery. Claronette spoke extensively about her love of clothes and fashion. Describing her style as old-school Jackie O, she said that clothes fit and look better on models in fashion magazines. She admired these "flawless" models and said they look "proper" and "orderly." However, this aesthetic ideal led to personal disappointment when she looked in the mirror and saw a reflection she described as "out of shape," with this body part and that body part "all out of place." To tame what she considered an unruly body, Claronette had abdominoplasty at age thirty-one.

Mass media images, whether in fashion magazines or on television, constantly remind her of what society values:

> Now I want the breast to be lifted. People do not understand that when you get older, you go back down. Now in the back of our mind, we still want to look good. Every time you look at the TV, beautiful bodies, this and that. . . . With me in my age, I don't want to look all wrinkled . . . because we don't look at it as beauty. We look at it as ugly.

With age and gravity taking their toll, Claronette is contemplating going under the knife again to have her breasts lifted. In her mind, and on the basis of her understanding of societal expectations, her breasts are now ugly. Pervasive images of this media ideal, then— whether of perky breasts, curves, or youth—create body insecurity, which in part motivates surgery. It is noteworthy, however, that even when participants conceded that cultural ideals shaped their desires, they were adamant that they were not using surgery to *radically* transform their bodies to embody these ideals. So at the same time that Claronette coveted the look of the models she described as taut and perfectly proportional, she also said she did not want to be "pencil thin." Being "big-boned," she could never envision herself being the same size as a typical fashion model and would just "love to be a size 12."

While participants spoke about a mainstream feminine beauty ideal, especially in terms of its desired features—for example, thin, shapely, and taut—several women of color we spoke with discussed the influence of ethnic ideals. Specifically, some Latina participants said they felt pressure to live up to Hispanic ideals of femininity, a finding consistent with extant research.[22] For example, Ana Marie, who identifies as Latina, had breast augmentation at age twenty-five. During her interview she talked about how her ethnic heritage shapes her views of her body:

> In Hispanic culture, they like curviness, and I think I let it get to me too much. I got too conscious about it. They think that you cannot be completely pretty if you don't have boobs. They even made a show about it, like a TV show about it. Yes, so there's a pressure to have boobs. . . . It was such an issue for me. It was all in my head because my husband, he liked me the way I was. He doesn't care about outward appearances, but I just . . . I hate it. I couldn't wear a bathing suit.

Even though she has a supportive spouse who appreciates her body, Ana Marie had a difficult time shaking off Hispanic ideals of femininity. She admitted to feeling quite insecure about her body, even saying that she "looked like a snake." She expressed concern that men laughed at her. While she feels she has a "good face," she augmented her breasts because she sees breasts as a defining characteristic of womanhood in Hispanic culture. She wanted to "have the whole package." In Chapter 5, we revisit Ana Marie's story. Despite believing she would be happier after surgery, she ended up feeling mostly regret, even disclosing that she wished she had not succumbed to cultural pressures.

Ashley, another Latina we spoke with, had breast augmentation at age twenty-two. She too said that Hispanic culture idealizes large breasts. However, Ashley made it clear that it was not this Hispanic ideal that shaped her decision to undergo cosmetic surgery. Rather, being born and raised in the United States, she said she was influenced by what she described as an inescapable "American ideal" that she believes is "everywhere." Similar to Ana Marie, she hoped that breast augmentation would allow her to feel feminine. Although she was scared to have cosmetic surgery, she felt she had to muster the courage to overcome this fear because she felt so trapped by her body. However, unlike Ana Marie, Ashley was ecstatic about her decision to spend $8,000 for, to use her words, "confidence," "peace of mind," and "happiness." Fitting in with this feminine ideal gave her relief. She no longer felt trapped. She felt free, even saying that surgery made her complete.

Regardless of the specific source of cultural pressure and despite insight that cultural ideals are media-constructed ideals, participants' actions suggest that cultural images matter. They do meaningfully shape how women think about their bodies and the choices they make about them.

Reaping the Rewards of Normative Femininity

Women who embody normative femininity reap psychological, social, and material rewards. People and institutions reward those who embody physical attractiveness ideals, and those who do not—like "overweight" people—miss out. Instead, they are subject to stigma, stereotyping, and discrimination.[23] Participants acknowledged that looking beautiful and young has a host of advantages. For example, Janet first turned to surgery in her forties and by age sixty-four had undergone two face-lifts, a tummy tuck, and breast augmentation. She is a media buyer who also owns a horse racing stable. As we sat in a café on a sunny summer afternoon in Southern California, she talked about how career concerns motivated her surgery. Being a media buyer meant she was "involved with media all the time [and had] to look the part." Her job put her in the public eye and she felt strongly that appearance was crucial for job success. Life, she said, would be "awful" without cosmetic surgery. It helped her not only with her career but also with meeting men and feeling better about herself. Janet believed that cosmetic surgery had few risks if one hired a competent surgeon. She praised her surgeon throughout our conversation and said she would be seeing him soon to have more work done on her chin, face, and eyes.

Similarly, Linda, a fifty-seven-year-old personal chef with Le Cordon Bleu training, initially said that we live in a youth culture. She then retracted that statement and said:

It's a teen culture. It's not even a youth culture anymore . . . You don't want to be a teen but you don't want people to necessarily know how old you are when you're applying for a job. . . . I hate to say this, and I'm not trying to play games, [but] you want to keep them guessing.

Linda had rhinoplasty at age twenty-six but continues to get injections, such as Botox, Restylane, and Juvéderm, to "keep them guessing." She uses cosmetic procedures, surgical and not, to help her look "softer" and "less tired." This is particularly important for her because she believes that society has an age penalty such that people over forty-five face discrimination. When talking at length about the lack of equal opportunity for those past the culturally constructed beauty prime, Linda states emphatically that she does not want to be a teen. Looking significantly younger is not her goal. According to Linda, aging well is about being in her fifties with softer features and a refreshed look. She and other participants thus turned to cosmetic procedures to keep them competitive and feeling good in a job market they feel favors youth and narrow conceptions of beauty.

Participants also emphasized the importance of appearance for dating, even believing that they might not be married if it were not for cosmetic surgery. Lorna, a thirty-three-year-old elementary school teacher who had facial surgery in her teens, spoke frankly about her current marital status. "Well, I know as a Christian I should say that God is my only man—or Jesus is—I get that. But for me, being asked out for the first time, I don't know. Would I be married? Would I have had the love experiences that I did?" This type of rhetoric can be attributed partly to how participants think potential partners perceive their bodies. Recall Ana Marie, who felt pressure to live up to ideals of femininity in her Hispanic community. She reflected, "I don't know if it was real or I made it up in my head, but I thought it was real. I thought men laughed about my body because they thought I looked like a little girl." Barbara, who had lost a large amount of weight after weight loss surgery, was concerned about how men would react to the excess skin and fat on her lower abdomen. "It felt like an extra appendage to me that I needed to be rid of. . . . I was also really concerned about dating and what that would mean. If I should meet someone and want to become intimate with them, how would they react to it?" At age fifty-two, she had a trunk lift.

Similar to how individuals of size sometimes sense that strangers are judging them in public settings even if they may not be,[24] participants expressed fear that a "generalized other"[25] (who represents society's norms and expectations) might also be judging their perceived failure to live up to beauty standards. As their statements show, they articulated these fears as what-ifs. But these fears are in fact rational. They are consistent with research documenting stigma and discrimination against body and beauty nonconformists,[26] and they are often based on real experiences. Specifically, many of the women we interviewed told us that throughout their lives classmates, siblings, friends, parents, dates, and spouses teased and harassed them about their bodies. Several participants used the phrase "kids are mean" and illustrated it with their stories. Reese said that, in sixth grade, classmates called her the "president of the itty-bitty committee." She had breast augmentation at age nineteen. Classmates taunted Rebecca, calling her "Miss Piggy" and "pig nosed." At age nineteen, she had rhinoplasty. Jessica heard girls refer to her as "sailor's delight," "sunken chest," and "flat as a board." She had breast augmentation at age twenty. Ashley, who had breast augmentation at age twenty-two, recounted how callous classmates gossiped about her, saying, "What's wrong with her? . . . Someone needs to develop that girl," only to have another classmate taunt, "Oh, they can. It's called plastic surgery." Family members, too, were unforgiving. Lily grew up with a brother who would call her "witch nose" and a grandmother who said, "Whatever child [is] born with my nose, I'm going to help fund a nose job!" Thus a seed was planted at an early age that her nose was a problem and surgery a solution. At age twenty, Lily had rhinoplasty.

Participants turned to surgery not only to avoid this type of negative feedback but also to procure benefits. Caitlin's story exemplifies how women who undergo cosmetic surgery are culturally savvy and know there is a social hierarchy that stigmatizes and penalizes beauty nonconformity while prizing and rewarding beauty conformity. She obtained breast implants at age twenty-four when she was, as she said, a "very, very single mother." She described her background as "the lowest economic class you could think of." Her dad died when she was young, and her mom had a disability that prevented her from working. Growing up, there was no family car. She said that the family ate poorly and that it showed in her figure. Everything about her, she said, "screamed trailer park." When she reached her twenties, she felt as if she looked like "a bad forty, not a regular forty." In her eyes, she also had "a completely flat chest."

Caitlin had been with her child's father for almost twelve years when she noticed him admiring other women who, she said, "looked like girls." She reflected, "He should love me for the way I am, you know," and she described how she held onto this perspective during a "decade of misery." She finally realized, "You can either continue this way or you can do something about it," and the two eventually separated. As a new single mom she felt she needed to change her appearance to get ahead in life:

> I've never had a problem with my brain. It was a problem with my appearance and [how] society perceives you. And you get further in life if they perceive you positively. I had a goal, and [surgery] was the means to the end. The means to stability. A husband. Job. School. Everything. And I think having my daughter [living with me as a single mom] and realizing . . . "You're on your own. This isn't a game anymore. Somebody depends on you." You do what you gotta do. And so I used my student loans and got boobs.

While she laughed several times during our exchange, she was also quite serious. Her belief that appearance is critical for a single mom's social mobility was a key motivator. Caitlin turned to cosmetic surgery as a tool for increasing career and dating opportunities. It was her path to escaping a life of economic instability. She explained why, in her view, looks matter so much for success in life:

> Just think about it as [if] you're in a herd. Thinking about it as animals. Like, there are these monkeys, [and] . . . whoever got the brightest blue balls is the alpha. . . . When they fight and the one that loses, his balls aren't as blue anymore. . . . And

so when you have the nails, the eyelashes, and the boobs, and stuff like that, people listen. They listen more. They pay attention more. . . . Because you have to look at it from a biology standpoint. They're looking for the best possible mate. And they are programmed to look for that mate, and you can't take offense by it. They're looking for as alpha as they can get. As are we females. So, I mean, you have a choice. Do you want this male? Do you want to try to make yourself an alpha? Or do you just be a doormat for the rest of your life? And I was tired of being a doormat for so many people. So, um, yeah, it did compromise everything I believed in. But in the end I got what I wanted.

Drawing on arguments rooted in evolutionary psychology, Caitlin described her need to make herself more physically appealing to attract an acceptable spouse. At the time of her interview, she had earned a bachelor of science degree and was in the process of completing a master's degree. She had been married for seven months. She described her spouse as a stable and successful "alpha male" who treats her and her daughter well. He is educated and in a higher class than her. She beamed and said, "We'll never have to worry again."

In sum, participants used cosmetic surgery to align how they appear on the outside with their sense of self, to feel more feminine, and to achieve various outcomes. They embraced an empowerment narrative. From their vantage point, cosmetic surgery is a medical innovation that empowers women by allowing them to feel and look normal, in which *normal* is defined by hegemonic ideals of femininity.

Stigma, Social Networks, and Cultural Reference Points

Participants are motivated to embody normative femininity via cosmetic surgery. Yet this method of body modification can come with stigma. The body surgically altered in the name of beauty is subject to criticism. Participants are certainly aware of this, although their social networks and cultural reference points shape this awareness.

Participants' social location and the social networks they are embedded in influence the extent to which they perceive and experience stigma. For example, several participants in California explained that cosmetic surgery was commonplace in their social circles. Confirming the possibility of a new normative aesthetic of artificiality,[27] these participants (who are predominantly white and embedded in relatively privileged class networks) sense that cosmetic surgery is so commonplace that there may be stigma placed on those who do *not* have cosmetic surgery. Forty-year-old Rebecca, who lives in Southern California, said about her peers, "They're just trying to keep up, and they feel like everybody else is doing it, and they feel like now it's the odd ball [thing] not to do it." Rebecca regretfully admitted to feeling the same way.

When asked to comment on how she thinks others view cosmetic surgery, Heather replied that she felt they were used to it: "I don't know if that's because of our geography of where we live [Southern California] and the community that I'm around, cuz I tend to be around socially middle- [to] upper-class people. . . . Because it's so common, I think [we] have become accustomed to seeing it. And I think we begin to like what we're accustomed to." In Heather's circles, cosmetic surgery is common. And she reasons that people come to like what is common. She joked that the men she knows prefer a surgically altered aesthetic because they are so used to "seeing fake." She continued, "I'm like, 'Really?' I think natural is really pretty."

Other Californians discussed the mainstreaming of cosmetic surgery and how beauty obsession is widespread. Lena described Orange County (OC) as "the worst." She is a divorced stay-at-home mom raising two teenage boys. She joked that she is grateful she does not have to raise girls in Orange County. Throughout her interview, she chatted at length about OC beauty culture. She had grown up in the area, and it was not uncommon for girls at the local high school to have cosmetic surgery, particularly to mark special occasions. "It's boob jobs for sixteenth birthdays and nose jobs." At age eighteen, dissatisfied with her nose, she did what her peers did. She asked her parents for a nose job as a high school graduation present. Choosing a surgeon was simple. Her mom had undergone two nose surgeries, breast surgery, and a face-lift. So she went with her mom's surgeon. Several years later and married, at age twenty-five, she had breast augmentation.

Lena described how she struggled with weight issues from early childhood and how living in Orange County resulted in her having "huge body image issues." Her parents exacerbated her low body esteem by holding her to high standards, whether it was about academic achievement or physical appearance. At a young age, she was put on diets and told she had to look pretty. Lena reflected, "It wasn't as awful like *Toddlers and Tiaras* or whatever, but it was very much like, there are expectations of grades, looks, and behavior." She believes her parents were primarily acting in her best interest: "They weren't these awful cruel folks. They just didn't want me to have the stigma of fat." Although she is an adult now, these cultural and parental pressures remain deeply engrained. At age forty-four, still living in Orange County, she continues to exhibit high body consciousness: "I am constantly aware of what I look like or what I wear."

At the same time that OC beauty culture places pressure on girls and women, it tempers the perception and experiences of stigma associated with cosmetic surgery. Thus, when asked if she thinks cosmetic surgery has a bad rap, Lena replied, "What's really funny is that I think it depends on which circles that you're in. I think around here, I think the average person probably doesn't think twice about plastic surgery." She continued to describe how her immediate social network consists of women who normalize cosmetic procedures, making them a part of everyday life:

> My friends are, like, other moms, like my kids' friends' moms and stuff. None of us are executives or fashion models or anything else. Everybody is doing everything they can to maintain, because it's really—I don't want to say competitive, but it's just like everybody is looking and judging around here. My two best friends, they just had a nose job and a boob job, and she gets filler and Botox. And my other girlfriend, she gets filler and Botox. She's got the perfect body. She's never had anything done to it. No, it's normal. I mean, like, someone says, "Oh, hey, I'm going to get Botox," [and everyone says,] "Oh, how is that?" "I want to do that." "Oh, I'm going to give you my doctor's name."

Lena points out that she is not an executive or a fashion model. As a stay-at-home mom surrounded by other moms, her environment consists of what she considers to be other average women, albeit women who normalize cosmetic procedures in a competitive beauty environment. While social judgment about physical appearance in Orange County may be harsh, the solutions, including cosmetic surgery, are widely embraced. A notable race and class element overlays these geographically specific perceptions. Lena is not only white; she is socioeconomically privileged. We revisit Lena's narrative in Chapter 5 because of her fraught relationship with cosmetic surgery.

Similarly, Marianne directly attributed having breast augmentation to living in Dallas and being embedded in elite circles. She is white, fifty-four, and holds a senior position at a bank. With an annual salary over $180,000, she clearly does not struggle to pay bills. She is poised, confident, and articulate. Unlike some participants who showed up to their interviews in casual clothing, Marianne arrived well dressed, manicured, and picture perfect. In fact, she mentioned during our conversation that she does not leave her house without wearing makeup, attributing this to growing up in a southern Mississippi debutante culture that emphasizes perfection.

Marianne's first cosmetic procedure was not planned. Growing up, she hated her "hooked nose" and was self-conscious about it. She wanted Cheryl Ladd's nose.[28] On Good Friday in 1979, a nineteen-year-old Marianne was driving home in her VW Beetle when a truck suddenly pulled out in front of her. Seconds later, her head went through the windshield. The accident, while horrendous, provided an opportunity. Luckily, she said, her nose was broken, and she had to have surgery. This early rhinoplasty in her teens was followed by liposuction and breast augmentation at age forty and a partial face-lift in her early fifties. These days Marianne's peer network consists mostly of successful women like her. She admits that being surrounded by women who have had breast augmentation influenced her decision: "There was a lot more pressure in Dallas." She continued, "I got a little bit more desensitized to—because everyone there—it was so acceptable, openly talked about. . . . That made it a lot easier to go, you know, there's no reason not to go ahead and do that."

Yet it is not only social networks shaped by geography, race, and class that affect meanings about beauty. Pervasive ideologies in ethnic communities also matter. As illustrated earlier, Hispanic beauty standards are meaningful to Latina participants, shaping body dissatisfaction and self-perceptions. We met Parvina, our only Middle

Eastern participant, in California when she was thirty-five—five years after she had rhinoplasty. At the time of the interview, she was a medical student. She was self-assured, light-hearted, and voiced strong beliefs about the subject matter. She focused the conversation quite a bit on Persian beauty culture and her view that criticism and perfection are pervasive in her culture:

> PARVINA: [My family is] very critical. Even if you touch one eyebrow, in my family, even one eyebrow out of line, oh my God. They know. It's like you're under a microscope constantly, and I think that's another fault in my culture. It's like, come on, be happy with what you are, but everyone always wants to strive for perfection, whatever their definition of perfection is. I'm still trying to figure that out. I'm not perfect, believe me. Not in my culture. With my weight? No way. Someone mentioned me getting lap band gastric surgery. I'm like, are you crazy? I'm surprised I don't have an eating disorder by now!
>
> INTERVIEWER: Do you feel that they put inordinate pressure on you?
>
> PARVINA: Yeah, it does. If someone is in your family, these are people that are supposedly protecting you, but it doesn't help, too. But when you go, like I was there in Iran, I had strangers telling me I was fat. And I'm a very outspoken person. Very brutal. No filter. So now I use sarcasm, and wit, to cut back, which is not good in my culture because you're supposed to be submissive, and so when I give it back to them, they shut up. They don't like it.

Persian culture, Parvina opined, patrols women's bodies and demands perfection, whatever that may be. She joked that she is surprised she does not have an eating disorder. While Parvina fights back with her sharp tongue and clever wit, she also admits to succumbing to cultural pressures by having rhinoplasty. Her sister and best friend have done the same. She continued to jest, "Everyone and their mother in the Persian culture have their nose done once, maybe twice!" Thus, similar to Lena's OC beauty culture, which exhibits both widespread beauty surveillance and widespread acceptance of cosmetic surgery, so too does this critical Persian culture Parvina describes. In both cases, alongside an oppressive beauty culture is a beauty work culture that situates cosmetic surgery as a normative solution for women and tempers the stigma typically associated with it.

Concerns about Stigma and Stereotypes

Despite evidence that cosmetic surgery is less stigmatized in some social circles, most of the women we spoke with—including those embedded in these aforementioned circles—still recognized and expressed concern that cosmetic surgery has a bad rap. So while being around others who have had surgery may serve as a buffer against social judgment, there nevertheless remains a pervasive cultural narrative that disparages cosmetic surgery and those who have it. As Ana Marie plainly put it, "The people that have surgery get judged by others, . . . and I think that's not fair." For example, participants acknowledged cultural stereotypes about people who have cosmetic surgery and were cognizant that others might judge them for having surgery that is considered unnecessary and a waste of money, is associated with vanity, and is connected with a failure of character.

Surgery as Unnecessary

Cosmetic surgery is elective in that it is scheduled in advance, done by choice to improve quality of life, and not required to address a life-threatening medical emergency.[29] The American Academy of Cosmetic Surgery recognizes this when it states that "treated areas, while lacking aesthetic appeal, function properly."[30] Participants acknowledged the elective nature of their surgeries and that others might see their decision as foolish because it involves unnecessary risk in the name of beauty. Sylvia alluded to how it is not socially acceptable to put oneself willingly in harm's way: "You're going to be in [an] operation. You could die. . . . If you don't have to go under the knife, you're not supposed to." Mothers, especially, had their share of misgivings about surgery, expressing concern for their children's well-being should something happen to them on the operating table. Leanne put it this way: "Here I go in, you know, to get something that's just totally unnecessary. And what if I don't wake up from the anesthesia? So that's kinda where my thoughts went. I mean, my daughter had her father, but he was a nonparticipant alcoholic parent." Leanne is forthright about the possibility of dying. She was aware she was taking what others might construe as an unnecessary risk and possibly shirking her responsibilities as her daughter's primary caregiver.

Precisely because it is elective, typical cultural norms about surgery are no longer in play. For one, cosmetic surgery is not considered a legitimate reason to take time off work. Kristen, who took time off to have cosmetic surgery, said in reference to her coworkers, "I was thinking they were thinking, 'This is what she's taking off work for? This isn't even a medical reason!'" Rebecca, who admitted she is "not proud" of her surgeries and finds it embarrassing to disclose them, remarked how cosmetic surgery is different from surgeries undergone for health reasons: "It's elective, so [others] can't really feel sorry for you." Unlike patients who undergo surgery aimed to preserve health and life, cosmetic surgery patients are not able to play the "sick role."[31] In the typical sick role, the person is not responsible for her condition and is consequently exempt from usual social roles and responsibilities. In contrast, women who have cosmetic surgery elect this stigmatized role, thereby negating the implicit rules about patient empathy and social responsibility. Social discourses suggest they should not be jeopardizing their obligations as mothers and workers in the name of beauty.

Surgery as a Waste of Money

Participants also acknowledged that others may pass judgment on them for wasting money. Take Roxanne, a fifty-year-old software consultant who grew up in Michigan and relocated to California. She underwent breast augmentation, which she did not disclose to her family members in Michigan. Back home, she said, it is a "huge thing" to spend money on cosmetic surgery. Illustrating the influence of social and geographic networks, she confessed that she might not have had surgery if she had stayed in Michigan because "it's not the focus [there]. It's just a whole different culture. A whole different mind-set . . . to spend money on that [cosmetic surgery] . . . was like, 'Wow, that's like $5,000!'"

Similarly, Kristen showed awareness that spending $11,000 on breast augmentation and an abdominoplasty is not a socially approved way of spending money. Her surgeon is mindful of this social disapproval and provides his patients with the option of putting his name on the cashier's check, rather than the name of his practice, which reveals his specialty. Kristen went this route, she explained, to be more discreet. She expressed concern that others would judge her. When asked to clarify how people might judge her, she said, "They think your priorities are backwards, like, 'Why would you spend all that money on plastic surgery?' . . . 'You know what I can do with that money?'"

In fact, some participants were told outright they wasted their money. Sylvia struggled after surgery to keep weight off. A relative chastised her, "See, you wasted all that money. There you go gaining weight." She said that, out of respect for his being an elder, she remained silent. However, she admitted to us, "I would like to answer, 'Well, you didn't pay for it, so don't worry about it.'" One participant's mom was also direct in her indictment. When Kristen asked to borrow fifty dollars, her mom replied, "Well, if you didn't spend all that money on your surgery, you wouldn't be in this situation." Kristen said, "They kind of throw it in your face. She's told me that on multiple occasions." Her mom's words point to disapproval of her daughter's choice to spend $11,000 on elective, and thus unnecessary, surgery.

Surgery as Fake, Superficial, and Vain

In American discourses, cosmetic surgery is about achieving beauty and sexuality ideals. It is associated with the rich, famous, and vain. Participants like Elaina voiced awareness of these stereotypes. She described the stereotypical cosmetic surgery patient: "You only do stuff like that [have cosmetic surgery] if you're wealthy or you have money." She stated that the image of the cosmetic surgery patient is that "she thinks she's all that. . . . She must have money. Yeah, those money people, you know how they are. They always want to look perfect. They have that belief . . . , that kind of stuff is only for the movie stars. 'Who does she think she is, a movie star?'" It is therefore unsurprising that participants expressed concerns that they would be characterized as, to use their words, "vain," "superficial," "artificial," "into looks," or a "sellout." For example, Kristen was concerned with accusations about superficiality: "They think you're bougie. They think you're shallow. They think you have your priorities backwards." Ashley, who disclosed her breast augmentation only to a small number of people, was uneasy that others would think, "Oh, she's so superficial. She's fake. That's stupid. . . . Or they're fake. Those are not even yours. They're plastic." Casey stated frankly, "There's a natural tendency to think that it's driven entirely by vanity." Or as Linda stated, the prevalent cultural sentiment is that those who get cosmetic surgery are into themselves: "Self-involved. Narcissistic." Simply put, participants are well aware of stereotypes that depict women who have cosmetic surgery as too heavily invested in their looks, frivolously spending large amounts of money on themselves in what is regarded as the selfish pursuit of beauty.

Surgery as Failure to Change through Socially Approved Means

There is a pervasive American ethos that people can transform their bodies as long as they try. For example, Americans generally believe that body weight is controllable and a function of self-determination and the Puritan work ethic.[32] People merely need to apply themselves if they want to change their bodies. This is captured in the long-running Nike slogan Just Do It!

Alongside this belief that individuals *can* transform their bodies, there is an expectation that they, especially women, *should*. Femininity and beauty are intertwined such that beauty is strongly mandated for women.[33] In a makeover culture, women are expected to discipline their bodies to adhere to normative beauty standards by, say, losing weight, shaving their body hair, wearing makeup, and more.[34] They are supposed to practice self-care. A commitment to care for and modify the body is considered a reflection of a strong ethos and moral fortitude, whereas a lack of commitment reflects a self that is wanting. Not living up to embodiment norms—whether intentional or not—is seen as a failure of the self and is thus subject to social sanction.[35]

Because the body is a reflection of the psyche, there are both acceptable and unacceptable means of transforming it. Acceptable means test an individual's inner strength, while unacceptable means are seen as cheating. For example, the socially acceptable way of achieving weight loss is tweaking the calories consumed versus calories burned equation. This involves monitoring food and beverage consumption and increasing physical activity levels. These means are deemed acceptable not only because they are the official stance of public health authorities[36] but because they supposedly reflect strength of character. Tweaking this balance requires discipline. Individuals must show restraint in their consumption behaviors alongside determination to increase their activity levels. Weight loss via these means involves patience and commitment to long-term goals, ostensibly reflecting strong moral fiber.

In this way, in public discourses, cosmetic surgery—and especially procedures involving the removal of fat tissue such as liposuction— are suspect. They can be interpreted as a form of cheating and failure to use socially approved methods to sculpt the body. Because the body is a reflection of the psyche, cosmetic surgery subsequently reflects a failure of the self. The woman who has cosmetic surgery has supposedly taken the easy route. Her aesthetic achievements purportedly do not reflect countless hours at the gym, the tedious counting of calories, and the forgoing of favorite foods. Instead, as Nadine said, there is the sense that "of course she looks good. She had a face-lift. She had lipo. She had a boob augmentation. [It's] cheating." Nadine disclosed that she is secretive about having had liposuction, and before her surgery she told coworkers vaguely that she "had something removed." She confessed, "[I felt] a kind of an embarrassment . . . that I couldn't get rid of it myself. Couldn't lose it myself."

Nadine's guilt likely stems from pervasive cultural sentiments that tell her she must sculpt her body through hard work. Similarly, Robin, who had a tummy tuck, described how others are quick to make assumptions about those who have cosmetic surgery: "There is a little bit of stigma with it, though. People who don't understand the process of it, they just think, 'Oh, it's a quick fix-it.'" Immediately after surgery Lacy was reticent to disclose she had liposuction for the same reason: "I really don't tell anyone. . . . They're going to think that I'm just so lazy." She elaborated:

It was the fear that people would be like, they would think I'm lazy. That I took the easy way. Where, you know, I imagine it's the same where someone gets bypass surgery or a lap band. And they're like, "Oh, well, you didn't diet or exercise. You went and just got the fat sucked out of you. Or you just got your stomach shrunk" or whatever. . . . But I didn't want to tell them 'cause I didn't want them to be like, "Why did you do that when you could try to take better care of yourself?" If someone asks me about it, I'd be happy to tell them. . . . But if we're not talking about it, it's not something I bring up.

While Lacy is not willing to lie about having liposuction, she voiced concern that others might think she is lazy or failed at self-care. In sum, participants were mindful that cosmetic surgery, particularly surgeries involving fat tissue removal, would be perceived as failure. They feared indictment on the grounds that they failed at body sculpting on their own through hard work and discipline.

Surgery as Failure to Accept One's Body

Ironically, at the same time that there is a pervasive ethos to change the body through socially sanctioned means, there are also widespread cultural discourses centered on self-acceptance, including body acceptance. For example, the National Organization for Women (NOW), founded during the second-wave feminist movement, has a long-running Love Your Body campaign. The campaign points out that women's beauty ideals are narrow, unrealistic, and often hazardous to women's health. In response, NOW encourages women to "be models of self-acceptance and love in front of young children and each other [and] support television shows and advertisements that show diversity and realistic versions of women."[37] Similarly, the Black Is Beautiful movement encourages black girls and women to embrace their natural features as beautiful.[38] Jessamyn Stanley exemplifies cultural discourses of self-acceptance. She is a black lesbian body-positivity advocate who teaches yoga. The subtitle of her book *Every Body Yoga* reveals her philosophy of self-acceptance: *Let Go of Fear, Get on the Mat, Love Your Body.*[39]

Corporations too have jumped on this love-your-body bandwagon. Dove, a soap brand, has a Self-Esteem Project,[40] and American Eagle, a clothing store, has advertised their Aerie line using plus-size models in unretouched photos.[41] This ever-growing body-acceptance movement in its many manifestations celebrates body diversity and encourages girls and women to embrace who they are. Notably, these cultural movements tend to condemn rather than promote cosmetic surgery. In fact, the Body Image Movement states that this movement involves "giving an alternative to cosmetic surgery, and learning to live and love your body."[42]

Surgery thus represents a second possible failure. Women who undergo cosmetic surgery potentially face another form of social rebuke. They have, purportedly, failed to accept their bodies. They allegedly lack self-esteem and confidence and have such poor body image and body security that they resorted to surgery. Charlize's statement at the start of this chapter captures how she feels judged for her "fake boobs." She expressed her overall concerns about the stigma of surgery:

When I'm on my back, they're there. They don't move. It's like a Barbie doll or something. So it's—if you have big boobs and they're natural, nobody can say anything to you. There's no judging. They can't judge you for having natural large breasts. But then when you go and get a boob job, it's different. It's like, oh, well, you have big boobs, you have fake boobs, but they're not natural. Then all of a sudden, it's just really funny because if you're born with them, there's no judging. But if you've gone and gotten them, then there's like this judging that happens.

When asked how others might judge, she replied, "It makes the person who got the boobs seem less real, less authentic. It's like, 'You're so insecure that you had to go get fake boobs. Why can't you be proud of yourself the way you are?'" Charlize is concerned that others might interpret her breast augmentation as a sign that she is inauthentic as well as insecure. It potentially reflects poor self-esteem and low confidence. As she put it, she should be proud of herself the way she is. Charlize is not alone in recognizing this indictment and failure of the self. Ashley's words capture what she believes is a common view people hold of women who have cosmetic surgery: "Why did you get that done? You should accept yourself for who you are."

Managing the Surgically Altered Body

Cosmetic surgery is an investment in the self. Feeling that they do not embody cultural norms of femininity, women turn to cosmetic surgery to achieve normative femininity and reap its rewards. However, they readily acknowledge that the body, surgically altered in the name of beauty, is open to judgment. Susceptibility to this judgment varies. Social networks—whether based on geography, class, race, or ethnicity—that place pressure on women to comply with beauty norms may also serve as a buffer to criticism when they do have surgery. Even so, participants exhibit an ongoing concern that they are permanently altering their bodies in a manner that is stigmatized and an indicator of failure. Cultural discourses paradoxically frame cosmetic surgery as a failure to both change one's body through praiseworthy methods and accept one's body. Yet not living up to cultural standards of beauty, particularly in a makeover culture, is also a source of stigma. Women who do not win the genetic lottery are essentially in a lose-lose situation. How, then, do they manage the cosmetically surgically altered body? What strategies do they use to preserve a valuable sense of self? The first step involves pursuing a very specific type of surgical outcome—the natural fake.

3

Pursuing the Natural Fake

> I wanted to come out looking like I have a natural-looking breast. That was all that mattered to me. . . . I didn't want people saying, "Oh, she's had a boob job."
>
> —ALLISON
>
> I know plastic surgery isn't natural. But you can make it appear so.
>
> —LILY

P articipants desired cosmetic surgery so they could look and feel more feminine and reap the rewards of normative femininity. However, they desired a specific type of surgery that met their expectations of what is acceptable. Specifically, they wanted natural results. But what exactly do participants mean by this? What are "natural" surgical outcomes? And after going under the knife, do they still consider their bodies natural?

The Desire for Natural: "Work Your Magic; Just Make Sure It Looks as Natural as Can Be"

Because participants are investing financially, sacrificing their physical comfort, and putting themselves at risk, first and foremost, they wanted to come out of surgery looking good. They expressed fears about scarring and permanent disfigurement and prioritized aesthetic outcomes. For example, Darla contemplated rhinoplasty for about four years and paid about $12,000 for the procedure. She stated bluntly her major fears: "Infection. Death. Unsatisfactory results." Jenna, who had rhinoplasty after thinking about it for "years," even placed aesthetic concerns above health concerns. Despite having

surgery in part to correct a deviated septum,[1] she said the appearance of her postoperative nose was more important than the prom-
ised health benefits of surgery: "My biggest fear . . . when they took
the bandages off was not that I couldn't breathe right but was the
way my nose was going *to look*. . . . I thought, 'Oh my God, what am
I going to do if the bandages come off and I hate my nose?'" This
fear of poor aesthetic outcomes was also manifest in participants'
disparaging of celebrities who had undergone surgeries they believed
resulted in unappealing outcomes.[2] Among those mentioned were
Pamela Anderson, Victoria Beckham, and Nicki Minaj. And in our
conversations we were asked several times about a specific American
reality television program: "Have you seen *Botched*?"[3]

Along with this fear of not looking good, participants had a desire for physical changes that look a certain way. Our conversations
revealed a recurring sentiment regarding participants' postoperative
bodies. This sentiment cut across racial, ethnic, and class lines. It
was also apparent across procedure type. It was the desire for natural
outcomes. Allison's chapter-opening quote captures this: "I wanted
to come out looking like I have a natural-looking breast. That was all
that mattered to me." Allison was thirty-two years old when she had
breast augmentation. It took her a year to commit to a surgeon. She
wanted to ensure that her surgeon could deliver breasts that would
look like they fit her body and would appear natural.

Allison was not alone in her desire for surgical results that appear
natural. Other participants prioritized this. They used the term *natural* or phrases that capture the same idea to describe ideal outcomes.
For example, Elaina said:

> I didn't want something to look fake. I wanted to look more
> natural. When I saw that it [rhinoplasty] looked natural on
> her [a friend who had cosmetic surgery], I thought, "If he did
> a good job like that with her, then he's definitely going to do a
> good job on me."

Similarly, Janet, whose surgical history includes face-lifts, a tummy
tuck, and breast augmentation, prioritized a surgeon who would give
her natural results. She spoke about several surgeons she did not hire:
"I didn't like the work they did. . . . You could really tell it was fake.

Their skin looked phony. They had those stretched-out, real tight—those lipo lips. They [the surgeons] wanted to do too radical." Meanwhile, Kerrie said, "I just wanted them [her postoperative breasts] to look very natural," while Lily explained:

> As with any good—I feel—cosmetic surgery, you want people to feel like something is different but not be able to tell what is different. So you don't want them to be like, tsk, you got a nose job! That wasn't on your face earlier. So you don't want to draw attention to that and I—people, when I say I had a nose job, they're like, oh, weird! It's not obvious to them. So therefore it makes me feel like it's natural.

According to Marianne, "I didn't want boobs that anybody would notice that I had boobs. . . . It was very important that mine did not look fake." Parvina expressed a similar sentiment, "I didn't want to have a snow slope [nose]. . . . [I said,] 'Do whatever you want to. Work your magic; just make sure it looks as natural as can be.'" And Reese stated, "I just wanted [my postoperative breasts] to look really natural." Participants' emphasis on the natural cannot be understated. It was a desire we heard time and time again. It was clearly important. For some, to use Allison's words, it was "all that mattered."

For some participants who had breast surgery, the desire for natural outcomes influenced the type of implant they chose. While there are several options for shape, texture, and feel, individuals contemplating breast implants typically choose either saline or silicone.[4] Through their own research, social networks, and surgeons, many learned that silicone implants more closely resemble the look and feel of natural breasts. Even the popular medical website WebMD states, "Many women say that silicone gel implants feel more like real breasts than saline."[5] For this reason, silicone sometimes held greater appeal. For example, Reese opted for silicone implants because, in her words, "I heard they felt more natural." Allison too wanted silicone implants because she believed saline "doesn't look as natural." However, because some participants perceived saline to be safer than silicone, even when they wanted the supposedly more natural look of silicone, they settled on saline.[6] The desire for natural-feeling and natural-looking breasts was also what motivated Charlize to go with implants over the muscle. Her surgeon told her, "If we go over the muscle, it allows the implant to fall with your breast naturally." In sum, participants hoped their new body parts would feel and appear natural. And they trusted their surgeons to achieve these natural results. Yet what precisely do they mean by this? How do they understand this term *natural*?

Conceptualizing *Natural*

God-Given and Unaltered

The adjective *natural* denotes something "existing in or formed by nature (opposed to artificial)."[7] Participants did not always use this exact wording, but in many ways their responses reflected this dictionary definition. They captured the essence of the first part of this definition—"existing in or formed by nature"—when they said a natural body is one that a person is "born with" or is "God-given." For example, when asked to describe the natural body, Ashley responded, "Natural flesh. Something that you'd be born with, like my natural hair, natural chin, [and] natural skin." Participants also stressed the latter part of this definition—"opposed to artificial." Natural bodies, they said, are untainted by human hands. "A natural body, it's just untouched," Kaylee said. Or as Casey explained, "It's letting your body look like it does without serious intervention." A body that is "untouched" or "without serious intervention" is opposed to one that is artificial. Certainly, both facets of the definition are related. If something is God-given, it is presumably untainted by artifice.

Participants explained that "untouched" or "without intervention" meant the absence of cosmetic surgery. A few even expanded their definition to include other forms of body modification. For instance, getting manicures and pedicures, dyeing hair, and using makeup could all be viewed as unnatural. Conceivably, by this understanding, anything but the naked human body would be considered unnatural! One participant also mentioned excessively working out at the gym and the use of anabolic steroids. What participants exclude from their conceptualization of natural, then, are actions that place the body on a trajectory beyond what they feel is the body's typical biological development. They seem to believe that bodies are born a certain way and then develop a certain a way. Human interventions that deflect the body from this "natural" developmental path result in a body they label "unnatural." The degree to which these interventions are permanent varies. On the one hand, nail polish, hair dye, and makeup are not generally long-lasting alterations. Cosmetic surgery, on the other hand, is.

Natural as Flawed

Such understandings of the term *natural* mean that participants inevitably see the natural human body as flawed. This is consistent with mass media's glorification of culturally compliant bodies. Most of us know that content in fashion magazines is highly staged, depicting female subjects who are immaculately groomed—from meticulously plucked eyebrows to flawlessly done makeup. Their bodies don cultural adornments—designer clothes and shoes—and their images have almost always been technologically altered using graphics software. They, participants agreed, are not natural. As Nadine, who works in computer graphics, said, "Well, it [natural] doesn't look like the models in a magazine. . . . No Photoshop." In fact, when public figures go au naturel, the event is deemed newsworthy. This was evident when the hosts of CBS's daytime talk show *The Talk* filmed the season 3 premiere without makeup.[8] Such an event draws attention to the cultural norm that dictates that women's bodies are not acceptable in their natural state. Mass media depictions, by default, implicitly convey the message that women's natural bodies are lacking. In response, women are prompted to buy advertised beauty products and services to transform their wanting, unaltered bodies into publicly presentable bodies.

Without human intervention, participants consider the natural body far from picture perfect. Nadine continued to describe the natural body this way: "It's got blemishes. It's got hair. Maybe a skin tag or two." Kristen added, "I would define it [as] droopy breasts, maybe a little stomach fat, legs kind of just there, there's not really much definition to it. That's what I think of when I think of a natural body. Arms just flabby, natural." Notably, Kristen's description of the natural body is rife with terms like *droopy* and *flabby*, which have a decidedly negative connotation. Similarly, when Casey compared unaltered breasts with surgically altered ones, she painted an unappealing portrait of the former. In her view, unaltered breasts are unattractive. They are also inconvenient and uncomfortable:

> The thing is, if women get breast enhancement, they're high, they're perky, and they're cooperative. Big natural boobs just go wherever they're going to go. They blob around . . . and they get pinned under things. They get twisted. They get pinched. Underwires poke in.

For Casey, unaltered breasts are neither "high" nor "perky." They are formless and "blob around." With age, she added, large natural breasts take a woman from "sex bot to matronly overnight." Drawing on personal experience, she concludes that large natural breasts are inferior to surgically enhanced ones.

In light of participants' understanding of the natural body as flawed, it seems incongruous that participants desire "natural" surgical results. The natural body is what they seem to be avoiding by having cosmetic surgery! However, a closer look reveals that naturalness and inconspicuousness are closely intertwined and that participants' understanding of what constitutes natural is, in fact, culturally constructed.

Surgically Inconspicuous: "Unless I Tell You I Had It Done, You Would Never Know"

Consider the perspectives of Lily and Lacy. Lily adopts the first part of the definition of *natural*—existing in or formed by nature. She had rhinoplasty at age twenty between her junior and senior years of college. She stressed that she "wasn't terribly unhappy" with her nose. It was just something she disliked and would notice, particularly in photos. However, because her parents were willing to gift her cosmetic surgery for her birthday, she moved forward with it. Lily was adamant that her surgeon understood that she wanted only a smaller version of the nose she already possessed. In her words, she wanted a nose that was not "so far from natural looking that it immediately attracts attention or people automatically feel like they know." After consulting with several surgeons, she met Dr. Matthews.[9] She sang his praises:

> So he had been doing it for a very long time, and he's known for doing discreet work because, um, he would be compared to doing the plastic surgery for the River Oaks moms. So if that makes any sense. In [the city where I had surgery] there's an old-money neighborhood, and he is their plastic surgeon. He is known for ... not just churning out huge Ds, button noses. ... He's crafted his skill; I guess it's more catered to the actual person and their look because those women want to be very discreet. ... Discreet, as in you can't tell so much that a woman had work done. Whatever look he was giving you, he wanted it to seem like it was something God could have blessed you with.

Lily describes Dr. Matthews as the surgeon of the city's social elites. Because she was hoping not to stray too far from the nose she was born with, he appealed to her. She felt he could create discreet results and not, as she said, a generic and obvious button nose. This would allow her postoperative nose to look like something she might have been born with. As she put it, her surgeon would be able to create results that seemed to be "something God could have blessed [her] with." According to Lily, "'Fake' to me is also the same as saying 'obvious.'" In her mind, natural surgical results are discreet and appear God-given—Lily's way of saying formed by nature.

In contrast, Lacy adopts the dictionary definition of *natural* as being "opposed to artificial." Lacy had liposuction on her stomach, thighs, and legs at age twenty, just after high school graduation and before starting college. She turned to surgery after struggling most of her life with her weight. As with Lily, her parents covered the cost of surgery. Although Lacy also contemplated having rhinoplasty and breast augmentation, she went through with only liposuction. She was concerned that, with the other two procedures, the surgeon was going to go "too big or too dramatic." She was comfortable with liposuction, knowing that "he's not going to take too much off, ... and it's very even, and he's very neat." She continued, "Liposuction was just more of a comfort place because it was like, 'Well, this is something that isn't going to change really the way that I look that couldn't be done naturally.'"

However, what does she mean by *naturally* here? According to Lacy, changing the body naturally means sculpting it through diet and exercise. Throughout our conversation, she chatted at length about how she struggled with both. She was not able to change her body through these "natural" means. Unlike Lily, who emphasizes that natural is what nature (i.e., God) might have blessed her with, Lacy emphasizes that natural is not artificial, meaning it is without human (i.e., surgeon) intervention. So while there are many ways to modify the body, Lacy hoped surgery would give her results that looked like they were achieved through what she considers natural methods, such as diet and exercise, and not unnatural methods, like cosmetic surgery.[10]

In both understandings—Lily's and Lacy's—of what constitutes natural, the desired results are inconspicuous. Lily said that *fake* means "obvious," and Lacy, with her surgery, wanted to avoid the dramatic. So whether surgery mimics the God-given or the nonsurgically achieved, the two women both desired inconspicuous results that blended in with their biological bodies. This end result does not reveal to the world that the body has been surgically altered. Thus, in the same breath that participants discussed natural results, they described results that would be, to use their words, "discreet," "modest," "conservative," "not noticeable," "not extreme," and "not overboard." This inconspicuousness is consistent with participants' desire (documented in Chapter 2) to blend in and be "normal." Parvina's words, which mirror Lily's earlier sentiment, show how participants conflate natural results with inconspicuous results: "In my opinion, when you do plastic surgery you're not supposed to do it to where it looks like you had it done; it is supposed to look natural. Unless I tell you I had it done, you would never know." This understanding closely resembles what researchers of other beauty practices observe. For example, research with Botox patients finds that aesthetic care "should be visually obvious, but not too obvious. . . . Women *should* use Botox, but they should not *look* 'Botoxed.'"[11] In the same way, surgical results should be an obvious aesthetic improvement, but they should not be an obvious surgical accomplishment.

In line with their belief that natural surgical results should inconspicuously blend in with their biological bodies, participants hoped to avoid unnatural results. The converse of so-called natural results includes the disproportionate, out of place, and most importantly, obviously surgically altered. Participants were especially critical of obvious breast implants. "Bad boob jobs," Lily said, are disproportionate and readily apparent to an onlooker. They look like what her dad calls "bolt-ons." Similarly, Reese was turned off by surgeon portfolios in which women appeared to have been given disproportionately huge breasts, "like watermelons." She said that, in the early stages of researching surgeons, she was looking for a surgeon who would allow her to "look really natural." Meanwhile, Marianne used the phrase "tits on a stick" to describe unnatural fake breasts, which were to be avoided at all costs. And Martha commented with an air of disgust, "I see a whole lot of women in this [Texas] town, and one of my daughters is like that. She's had a boob job, she's had all sorts of stuff. . . . Her boobs are too big, and she's starting to look duck-lipped. . . . I think it's awful."

Ironically, then, participants' goal was to look as though they did not have surgery. Research shows that surgically altered breasts are a form of conspicuous consumption to display upward mobility, but our participants steered clear of the "obvious fake."[12] Instead, they pursued the natural fake—a cultural achievement that disguises its very own presence. This natural fake serves as a defense against charges that one has done something worthy of criticism. As demonstrated in Chapter 2, participants are well aware of a wide range of charges aimed at people, especially women, who have cosmetic surgery. The natural fake, which is inconspicuous, protects them against these accusations. For instance, it shields them against charges that they have wasted their money on something unnecessary or accusations of vanity and superficiality. Or it shields them from allegations (overt or not) that they have undergone a type of surgery that public discourses frame as a failure of character.

By seeking and subsequently embodying the natural fake, they can now meet cultural standards of feminine beauty and blend in as surgically unaltered. This is likely why so many participants insisted that others could not tell they had surgery. Allison explained, "I didn't want people saying, 'Oh, she's had a boob job.' And most of the time, people don't know." According to Jasmine, "Nobody can tell. He did a good job. Nobody can tell they're fake." Marianne said, "It was very important that mine did not look fake. And they don't." According to Penelope, "They look very natural. I mean, you probably couldn't tell. They're very natural. My doctor—I go in for my annual physical. [She says,] 'What? Do you have breast implants? No!' It's like, yeah! [*laughs*]." Kristen spoke similarly of her changes: "They would never think in a million years that I had plastic surgery. It just looks natural." Parvina explained, "I've had people say, 'You shouldn't have [had] it done; we don't notice any difference.' I'm like, 'That's perfect; that's exactly what I want.'" Kerrie made a comparable statement: "A lot of people can't even tell that I've gotten them done, which is great." Elaina specifically credits her surgeon for results that are difficult to pinpoint as surgically altered: "[My friends] kept looking at my face, and they were like, 'What'd you do? You did something.' They kept looking at my eyes, my hair. They just couldn't figure it out. At that point, I was like, 'Wow, he's [the surgeon is] good.'"

Participants expressed delight that family members, friends, and strangers were in the dark. Kerrie, who opted for silicone gummy bear implants because she felt they were more natural,[13] was nervous about seeing her mom after surgery. When they finally met up, she was surprised by her mom's reaction. Apparently, her mom did not know: "She was like, 'What do you mean you got boobs?'" Kerrie took credit for her mom's obliviousness: "I got them natural enough to where you can't really tell." She was thrilled, she said. Similarly, Marianne shared a story about a conversation she had with several men, including one she was dating, about cosmetic surgery. The men openly stated they would never date a woman who had breast augmentation. With a wry smile, she said, "You are."

Downplaying Implants: Body Parts That Fit

Ensuring that one looks natural, and like one had not undergone surgery, manifested itself in a very specific way for participants who had breast augmentation. Several participants emphasized that their postsurgical breasts were not very big. For example, Marianne (who increased her bra size from a full A to a full B) said of her implants,

"I didn't want boobs that anybody would notice that I had boobs. So I wanted small boobs! [*laughs*]." Like Marianne, Heather (who increased her bra size from mid B to small C) downplayed the size of her implants. "I still added a B, small C. That's not big." Kerrie (whose bra size went from 32B to 32D) rejected her surgeon's implant size recommendation. She ended up going with smaller implants because she was concerned it would not look natural on her. Even Jasmine, who is 5'4" and 128 pounds and went from "just skin and a little breast tissue" to double Ds, insisted that she looks proportionate. She remarked that she does not look like "Dolly Parton" and is not "cartoonishly huge."

Grace, who augmented her breasts with silicone implants, chose her desired breast size of 32C because she thought it was about the average breast size in America. She is actually off the mark here. While studies estimating women's average breast size do have measurement problems, a 2013 survey puts the average for American women at 34DD, up from 34B twenty years ago.[14] Nevertheless, for Grace, this information influenced what she was looking for in her postoperative breasts:

> I guess just not having any abnormalities or looking too dramatic. You see a comic character. They have double Ds and a tiny waist. I've looked up what Barbie would look like if she was a real human. That's not real. I think just natural is just keeping it in those common denominators.

Again, the same language surfaces. Grace wanted to avoid breasts that do not look real. She wanted natural breasts. She did not want anything "too dramatic." She opted to increase her breast size from 32B to 32C, thereby keeping within "common denominators." Grace also believed that getting extremely large implants increases the risks associated with surgery. As she put it, because she "was going the natural route, [she] had the lowest risks." She admitted that there are days she wishes she had gone with larger implants but then stops herself from going down this path: "Sometimes I wish I went a little bigger, but then I'm like, no, because it wouldn't look natural then. . . . I would regret it if I got any bigger."

Participants' desire for discreet breasts also emerged in their advice for others contemplating surgery. Several women who had breast surgery warned others not to go too large and to stay within a few cup sizes of their current size so the outcomes would look natural. Grace has several friends "who are A cups" and are "saving up" for surgery. She said, "I wouldn't recommend them to go more than a full B because you don't want to look like Victoria Beckham, like two watermelons on a stick." Kaylee was especially dismissive of women who want extremely large breasts: "It wasn't anything too drastic for me. I'll say to someone [who is also considering implants], like, 'Okay, cool.' Unless they get super big boobs. I'm just like 'Why? That's completely unnatural!'"

Participants who had breast augmentation also said that their new breasts fit their body frame or structure. Along with "fitting," participants described them as "proportionate," "balanced," and "symmetrical." Right after Heather said her breasts were not big, she added, "I think it fits my frame." Marianne said, "If you look natural, you don't look like you've had surgery [*laughs*], which is my goal. It's sort of having that proportioned figure or look, the symmetry, I think." Roxanne also stressed balance: "My real motivation [was] just to look good and balanced, not to catch anybody's eye or anything like that." Hanna said that after breast augmentation surgery she felt sexier and beautiful and "more proportionate." Jessica, who like Grace admitted there are days she wishes she had chosen larger implants, nevertheless said that she is glad she did not go bigger: "I'm very pleased . . . because I'm for proportion. I still err on the side of conservatism." Ultimately, participants consider their postoperative breasts inconspicuous. In their view, they are proportionate and fit their bodies, reflecting symmetry and balance.

Feminine Enhancement and Restoration

As we point out in Chapter 2, the embodiment of normative femininity is a major motivator, and participants expressed a desire for breasts and curves to look and feel feminine. Here we add the criterion of the natural fake—that these artificially achieved feminine body parts be inconspicuous. In this way, participants viewed their surgeries as merely enhancements of the female form. (They also used the word *refinement*.) Kristen was especially vocal about this point. She felt that cosmetic surgery has an undeserved bad rap. She described how she and a friend who also had breast surgery wanted to only "enhance" their bodies. "We didn't want these crazy sculpted bodies that people thought were fake." She carried on, "We didn't look crazy. We wanted to just enhance ourselves." In her ideal world, aesthetic surgery would not be called "plastic surgery." Her preference would be "enhanced surgery." This would redirect the focus from *plastic*—a term that connotes artificiality and has negative meanings—to *enhancement*—a term that conveys subtlety and beauty and calls to mind naturalness.

Cosmetic surgery "enhancements" also serve a restorative function. Although participants voiced little desire to look like their teenage or twenty-something self, surgery still provided them a mechanism for turning back time. For example, women who had children said that pregnancy had stretched their stomachs, while nursing left them with what they felt were unsightly breasts. They turned to cosmetic surgery to restore their prepregnancy bodies. Sarah, now age thirty-eight, said, "I was a new mommy, my daughter was two or three at the time. I had breastfed. . . . I wasn't the same [woman] I remembered before my pregnancy." Cosmetic surgery, she maintained, "restored my sense of youth and put my body back to what I remember." Such restoration is presumably inconspicuous because one is only returning the body to a previous state on its developmental trajectory.

Similarly, participants who had face-lifts believed that natural surgical outcomes enabled them to restore something that was taken from them. However, here it was not pregnancy but aging that "damaged" their bodies. So when we asked Marianne, age fifty-four, if she felt surgery gave her a *new* face, we were politely corrected: "No, I felt like I was going back to my old face [*laughs*]. I felt like I looked like I did five years previously. . . . I went back to the same face, just improved. But once again, not a lot of people noticed." She is quick to point out that not only is she returning to her younger face but that she now embodies a successful natural fake; almost nobody notices she went under the knife.

Penelope was also keen to convey that cosmetic surgery is not about creating a new body. For her, cosmetic surgery is about preservation and restoration:

I look at it as more like preserving what you have. It's more like I'm trying to preserve, cuz I didn't always have saddlebags.

I mean, that came with age. You get a little older and start plumping out. And there it went, and I couldn't lose it. So it was like, give me back what I had. And same with the breasts. I mean, give me back what I had.

She continued to talk about how a skillful surgeon allowed her to look natural, the way she looked over a decade ago: "And all he did was, like, take me back about fifteen years. This was what I looked like fifteen years ago. . . . And that was very natural cuz that's exactly what I looked like. So yeah, I do think of myself as natural." She was sixty-one at the time of her interview. Worth highlighting is that Penelope believes two things about her postoperative body. First, she believes she looks natural because all her surgeon did was recapture her midforties' appearance. Second, and related, she still thinks of her body as natural despite having undergone multiple surgical interventions.

Postoperative Bodies

I'm Still Natural: "It's Just a Better Version of Me";
or, Nothing "Foreign" Added

Some participants saw their postoperative bodies and body parts as natural; others did not.[15] On the one hand, the absence of obvious change meant that, in their minds, postoperative bodies resembled preoperative bodies, only better—enhanced or restored. So participants such as Penelope and Marianne continued to see their bodies as natural, stressing that they still looked like their younger selves. Others, like Martha, emphasized the absence of anything dramatic. Recall, she was critical of women, including her own daughter, who had obvious implants. So when Martha was asked if she thought of her body as natural, she replied affirmatively, maintaining it was because she was "not overdone." The natural fake, which is inconspicuous, enables participants to frame their bodies as natural.

A number of participants who had liposuction, abdominoplasty, or rhinoplasty did not rely exclusively on this rhetoric of inconspicuousness. Instead, they also turned to a lack-of-artifice rhetoric. By focusing on the absence of an artificial object, they justified their bodies as natural. In their view, they have only shaved, sculpted, or removed. They have not *added* anything "foreign" to their bodies. A foreign object, they maintained, would increase the chances of surgery looking conspicuous. Implants, participants said, are "artificial." For example, Lavanna had abdominoplasty. She distinguished surgeries that involve removing parts of the body from surgeries that involve inserting something into the body. She refused to use the label *plastic surgery* for her abdominoplasty. In her mind, the logic is simple: "It's not really plastic surgery [when] you're just taking away something." She continued to say that, after nursing three boys, losing breast tissue, and feeling that her breasts are not as full, she is now thinking of having breast surgery. Unlike her abdominal surgery, which allows her to still be natural, she believes adding implants would make her body unnatural. This is her logic:

> If I get the breast implants, that is not natural. To me, that's more plastic surgery than what I had, because you have to keep that up. You have to go get them checked, you have to keep that up. The stomach is done. I don't have to go in for checkups and see if it's right. But when you have breast implants, you put something in the body that's foreign. So you do have to get that checked regularly to make sure everything is right. It's maintenance. 'Cause [getting a tummy tuck is] no different than getting a nose job. You get it done. You probably never have to worry about that again. You're not adding to it.

For Lavanna, removing fat tissue does not constitute cosmetic surgery, so the body stays natural. In contrast, a body that has an implant *has* been subject to cosmetic surgery and is thus unnatural. It now requires regular upkeep. With a tummy tuck or nose job, after the recovery period is over, one supposedly continues on the same life course trajectory one was on before surgery. The body may have experienced temporary trauma, but it returns to its previous physical state, albeit aesthetically altered. The worry supposedly also dissipates. In contrast, implants are foreign and therefore place the body—psychologically and physically—on a new and unnatural trajectory. There is potential "worry," and one must now have checkups to ensure "everything is right."[16]

Claronette and others expressed a similar view. She had undergone abdominoplasty and at the time of her interview was contemplating dental veneers. She said, "Now, I would be considered a fake
if they put something in me that wasn't there before." Susan, who had
abdominoplasty and liposuction, remarked that she was natural but
said, "I think what I would consider unnatural would be breast implants, chin, lip . . . because they're actually implanting stuff in your
body, or adding to. I'm just removing." Elaina, who had ear surgery,
talked about a friend who suffered burns to his face. He had "ears
put on." She then remarked, "That, I would consider unnatural. Even
though they look like they're his, but they're not his. For me, I'm
natural. . . . You don't have any other kind of implants, then you're
natural. Once you start getting implants, then you're not natural."
And Parvina, who had rhinoplasty, said, "I consider my new body
part natural because they didn't add anything, they just shaved. They
nipped, they tucked, and they shaved. They didn't add anything. So
I don't have to worry about that. I just feel it's a new, revised . . . me;
it's just a better version of me!" Like Lavanna, Parvina explained that
adding parts can create complications. Her nose surgery sans implant meant she did not fret about potential complications. During
our interview she talked about how breast implants are foreign to the
body and have the potential of leaking. She then described what she
thought was a "brilliant" procedure that allowed one to stay natural: "They will take your liposuction from [your] torso, and they will
inject it back into different body parts that need it to fill them out. I
think it's excellent. I think it's a very smart way of redoing something
that you needed. I don't think that's unnatural; I think that's perfect!"

I'm No Longer Natural: "I Know Plastic Surgery Isn't Natural, but You Can Make It Appear So"

Some participants maintained they were natural because they merely
enhanced or restored their bodies or because they did not put anything artificial in their bodies. A number of other participants, however, stated they could no longer refer to their bodies, and new body
parts, as natural. Consistent with their definition of a natural body
as one without serious intervention, they described their bodies as al-

tered. Taylor, who had liposuction, said she is not natural because she would not look the way she does if not for cosmetic surgery: "I know that if it wasn't for the surgery, it [my body] wouldn't be sculpted the way it's sculpted. Before, it was just straight, and now . . . I have a waist and I have a form. Before it was just body all over the place. It's not natural." Kristen who, as we pointed out earlier, was extremely vocal that surgery be about discreet enhancement and natural results, made a comparable point: "My body is definitely sculpted. It's been put together. It's like my breasts, my tummy. They kind of sculpt your hips. They give you more of a hip figure. . . . It's not natural. People aren't born like this. Come on now!" Kaylee too said her body is no longer natural: "Not anymore. I mean I know and I accept that I have implants and then I'm not completely natural." However, she goes further to emphasize a sentiment we heard repeatedly in some form or another: "I'm not saying I look unnatural. . . . I don't." Again, the natural fake with its *appearance* of naturalness is the benchmark. This is clearly captured in Lily's chapter-opening statement: "I know plastic surgery isn't natural. But you can make it appear so."

In sum, while the majority of participants insisted that their postoperative bodies are still natural, a handful voiced the opposite view. Yet those in this latter category still prided themselves on not *looking* as if they had been subject to surgical intervention. The natural fake is at its core about inconspicuousness.

The Natural Fake as a Cultural Construct

Participants view the natural body as culturally and biologically imperfect. It is problematic and must be tamed. With surgery, they hope to transform problematic body parts ("flab," "sagging lines and jowls," and "droopy breasts") into culturally acceptable parts (taut abdomens, tight facial skin, and voluminous and perky breasts). Yet successful cosmetic surgery that embodies the natural fake means not only altered body parts but postoperative body parts that are not radically different from what people are born with, could have been born with, or could have achieved through "natural" methods such as exercise and dietary changes. These postoperative parts are able to pass as God-given. In participants' eyes, the successful natural fake maintains proportion, symmetry, and balance with their God-given bodies. Surgery is refinement, enhancement, or restoration of their feminine form.

In reality, then, when participants embody the natural fake, they embody culturally sanctioned appearance norms. So even when they say they want to look natural, the natural here is more rhetorical than substantive. Substantively, the natural fake follows hegemonic and socially rewarded beauty scripts that are celebrated in mainstream media. If nature dictates a body's usual developmental trajectory, including aging and life course events such as pregnancy and breastfeeding, participants deliberately veered from this path and fought signs of these biological processes. Their description of the natural— as God-given, free of cultural intervention, and unruly—is really not their desired postoperative vision. Instead, their vision is of inconspicuous results that conform to cultural notions of femininity and youth. In fact, given how extreme it is to have surgery, there is an expectation that postoperative results epitomize cultural ideals. As Rebecca commented, "Oh, your boobs better be perfect tens. . . . Well, you paid for them. You went to a plastic surgeon; they better be perfect." The natural fake is thus the ultimate embodiment of cultural ideals.

Passing and Redefining

Passing is the process of presenting oneself as a member of a social category that one is not a member of.[17] It involves strategies of impression management that allow an individual to hide a stigmatized or discredited identity.[18] Within the context of cosmetic surgery, scholars have written about how cosmetic surgery enables women to pass as "normal."[19] Meanwhile, historians and social scientists have documented how cosmetic surgery can be used to facilitate racial or ethnic passing.[20]

Here we focus on how the natural fake enables passing. Because a body surgically manipulated in the name of beauty can be stigmatized as deviant, participants desired natural postoperative outcomes—an inconspicuous natural fake that conforms to hegemonic ideals of femininity. This natural fake allows them to pass as surgically unaltered and therefore avoid or minimize negative social repercussions. Consistent with other forms of passing, many participants were private about their surgeries. While some were open about their surgeries—often saying that this candidness was part of their overall personality—few participants publicized them. They disclosed their surgeries only to select friends and family members. Passing also meant hiding visible signs of surgery. Participants used creams to fade scars and positioned clothing strategically to cover evidence of having gone under the knife. These types of management strategies are the focus of Chapter 5.

Participants' understandings of *natural* enable them to frame their postoperative bodies as natural. This is because they consider their bodies as only slightly enhanced or restored. Or they said that their postoperative bodies did not contain anything artificial. In the absence of an artificial object, their bodies were not put on an atypical physiological and psychological path that involved, say, ongoing follow-up appointments or worry about complications. Moreover, even when participants felt they could no longer consider their bodies natural, they stressed the quintessential attribute of the natural fake—inconspicuousness. Those unwilling to embrace the rhetoric of having a natural body emphasized instead that, at the very least, they did not *look* as if they had been subject to surgical intervention.

In these ways the natural fake makes it possible for women to manage the cosmetic surgery paradox. They are able to pass as surgically unaltered and avoid social condemnation. They can also ward off charges of artificiality; their bodies are still natural or, at a minimum, do not look fake. However, the natural fake is more than a physical disguise that helps avoid charges of aesthetic artificiality. Rather, it is part of a larger package of boundary work that allows cosmetic surgery patients to preserve a gendered, authentic, and moral self.

Setting Boundaries

My breasts are fake, but I'd be like, "Do I look like a porn star to you?"

—Kaylee

I was adamant I was about not looking like a river rat woman.

—Leanne

In their pursuit of the natural fake, participants expressed disapproval of outcomes that appear unnatural. Bad cosmetic surgeries, they said, look "fake," with poorly altered breasts looking "cartoonish," like "watermelons," "bolt-ons," and "tits on a stick." By exalting the natural fake and condemning its antithesis, participants symbolically distance themselves from women who look "artificial." They effectively engage in boundary work—discursive practices by which individuals draw rhetorical, symbolic, and moral boundaries to distinguish themselves from others.[1] In fact, participants' exaltation of the natural and denigration of the fake was the most common form of boundary work that surfaced in our interviews. It was a prevalent theme that crossed class, racial, and ethnic lines. It was also evident across procedures.

Yet we observed other forms of boundary work. The boundary work participants exhibited ranged from accounts that their surgeries were necessary to accounts that good surgeries, like theirs, have good motives. Thus, in this chapter, we build on extant research showing that cosmetic surgery patients separate themselves from "surgical others," both real and imaginary.[2] According to the sociologist Debra Gimlin, surgical others are individuals (mostly women) who have a problematic, and sometimes pathological, relationship with cosmetic surgery. They are people who have had cosmetic surgery, whom participants may or may not personally know (e.g., friends, celebrities), and whom participants discredit. By distancing themselves from certain types of surgeries and certain types of people who have surgery, participants justify their own decisions and surgically altered bodies. Here we extend current knowledge by showing how boundary work processes involve retaining a gendered, authentic, and moral self. Specifically, good surgeries do not constitute a woman's entire being. Instead, they allow her to preserve a sense of self that, in her mind, is true to her self, moral, and not preoccupied with sexuality. Thus, despite participants' postfeminist rhetoric, the sense of self they seek to maintain through boundary work aligns with traditional notions of femininity.

Elective Surgery as "Necessary"

Our interview guide contained a question that gauged the extent to which participants felt surgery was life changing. We asked, "What do you think life would have been like without surgery?" Rather unexpectedly, most participants speculated that their lives would not have been much different. Sure, surgery made life better by allowing them to feel more physically attractive and confident. However, most surmised that they would be on the same life trajectory. For example, participants who went to college, got married, and established careers speculated that they still would have accomplished these things. Surgery was not viewed as life transforming. Instead, by increasing self-esteem and confidence, it made them a little more content in their life. For the majority, it was not a prerequisite for happiness.

There were a few exceptions. As reported in Chapter 2, Caitlin felt surgery was needed to thwart a life of poverty. Voluptuous breasts, she believed, would help her obtain an "alpha man" and facilitate social mobility. Ashley too viewed surgery as a game changer. Because of her high levels of self-consciousness, she felt she would still be "trapped" in her body had she not had surgery. With breast augmentation, she was finally "set free." And before her trunk lift, Barbara felt stuck behind a "wall of fear," even conjecturing that she would not be married without it. A small group of women believed surgery altered their lives dramatically, delivering emotional relief. They considered surgery necessary.

At the same time that most participants said surgery was not necessary for happiness, they framed surgery as necessary in another way. In line with one sociologist's observation that elective facial surgery can be reframed as necessarily lifesaving,[3] participants reframed cosmetic surgery as necessary, even though it is never technically needed to save their lives. Specifically, they pointed out that some body parts are immutable and cannot change without a surgeon's knife. The breasts and nose one is born with, they said, are beyond one's control. Consequently, if they are to be good female citizens, they "need" cosmetic surgery. Beauty discourses create a social backdrop pressuring women to live up to cultural standards of beauty, and makeover discourses beseech women to better themselves. The framing of surgery as necessary is a form of boundary work that allows women to justify cosmetic surgery and at the same time demonstrate concerted efforts at self-improvement in a social milieu that expects this of them.

For example, participants said that only surgery can correct uneven, small, or sagging breasts. Heather said, "I don't think that fake breasts are pretty. I feel like mine are a necessity. I'm glad I have them. I don't want to be without them. My first preference would be to have even, nice-sized shaped real breasts, but I don't have that option." By saying she does not have the option of having "real breasts" she finds attractive, Heather implies that she *must* turn to surgery, making clear that she believes in the beauty mandate and is willing to go under the knife to satisfy it. Other participants indicated that, while weight loss may result in a reduction of fat tissue in the breasts, surgery is the only way to increase breast size. Grace took a lighthearted stance when she said, "I have been twenty pounds heavier and my boobs did not grow any bigger. It went straight to my butt. . . . It's funny. It's like, man, even if I gain a lot of weight they're still not going to get bigger! The only thing to do was to get surgery." She plainly felt no other path was available. Hazel, who had rhinoplasty and breast augmentation, made a similar point while simultaneously stressing the futility of behavioral modification. In her words, "There are certain things you *need* cosmetic surgery for. Exercise is not going to fix my breasts ever!" Remarkably, Hazel is a full-time personal trainer and nutrition counselor. She has told clients they "needed a tummy tuck," saying there was nothing more she could do for them as a fitness professional. Like Heather, Grace, and Hazel, many participants told us that surgery was their only option. In these cases, biology limited their ability to reach their appearance goals. Rhinoplasty patients had similar views—only surgery can change a nose with which one is born.

Participants who had liposuction or abdominoplasty articulated a similar perspective. This is somewhat perplexing, because prevalent cultural discourses maintain that individuals can and should achieve weight loss and body sculpting through behavioral changes alone.[4] It soon surfaced that they framed these procedures as necessary only after making concerted efforts to modify body parts through culturally sanctioned means. They described long-term and repeated efforts to alter stomach, hip, and thigh areas via exercise, sports, dieting, and changes in eating habits. Despite seeing some visible changes, such as weight loss, they deemed these changes inadequate. Consider the words of some of the participants whose surgical histories include liposuction or abdominoplasty. Claronette said, "I just saw the ugliness of my stomach. I exercised, I walked, I did everything to try to flatten it back down, but I could not do it." Marianne explained, "I was small, but I always had those saddlebags. No matter how skinny I got, I couldn't—I was a size 2 or a 0—but I had fricking saddlebags." Nadine said, "I've always had this tummy, and I work out a lot but just could never get rid of it." Penelope told us, "Do what you can first. There is nothing you can do about a stomach that has been stretched out and gone back and forth. You lose the elasticity. . . . if you have a bump on your tummy that you just can't ever get rid of, liposuck it." And Taylor explained:

> I would cry in dressing rooms because I would try on clothes and they did not fit me. I would put pressure on myself because I was doing everything I needed to do. I've never been the type of person to be unhealthy. I was very active, and I had accumulated fat. I did things in high school, but it was fat that was just thick and not going anywhere. That was frustrating to me

because I put blame on myself. Once I did this [liposuction], now it's almost like I don't even think about that. Those problems are gone.

Participants' laudable efforts generated limited returns that made surgery, from their standpoint, not only reasonable but necessary. Their efforts also point to the limits of body sculpting—a reality that is overshadowed by pervasive cultural sentiments that emphasize the power of behavioral modification. Even Hazel, the fulltime personal trainer and nutrition counselor, conceded that there are limits to what one can accomplish through diet and exercise alone.

Taylor's self-blame is noteworthy. It reflects an internalization of the common cultural ideology that she can and should sculpt her body via physical activity and dietary changes. She described what some health experts might label an ideal lifestyle. Taylor goes to the gym four to five days a week to lift weights and participate in activity classes. When asked about her eating habits, we discerned a vigilant health consciousness. She admitted to having a sweet tooth, which meant having something like chocolate, ice cream, or popsicles after supper, but she otherwise ate healthily. A typical breakfast was eggs with vegetables such as asparagus or spinach, wheat toast, and coffee. Lunch and suppers consisted mostly of lean meats, fruits, and vegetables. Taylor's self-blame seems pretty harsh given that she follows the standard formula of monitoring calories going in and ensuring that calories are burned. She was noticeably frustrated that, in spite of her healthy lifestyle, the fat "was not going anywhere." Only with cosmetic surgery did Taylor achieve the results she was seeking, as well as experience emotional respite.

Surgeons are collaborators in this type of boundary work. They reinforce the message that certain body parts cannot change without their skillful hand. For example, Lavanna, who had abdominoplasty, said, "[My] doctor said [that] no matter how much exercise you do, that amount of loose skin is not going to tighten up." The surgeon Marianne hired for her liposuction distastefully claimed that even prisoners in concentration camps had saddlebags. She recounted her consultation: "And the doctor was like, 'Look, even in Auschwitz, as people were dying and being starved, they still had saddlebags, because if that's where your body stores its fat, that's where it's going to

store its fat.'" No doubt, these surgeons' words provide powerful am-
munition to combat the ubiquitous just-try-harder mentality. Even if
this message is self-serving, their words provide medical legitimacy
to support participants' views that they have done all the right things
before turning to surgery.

Consistent with this effort-first-surgery-second ethos, participants admonished others who turned to surgery too quickly. Indeed,
boundary work is about separating oneself from others, particularly
those one considers worthy of judgment. For example, Jenna, who
had rhinoplasty, stressed the importance of diet and exercise and
chastised those who do not make lifestyle changes before having surgery. In her words, "People want a quick fix. . . . The medical industry
makes it so easy for that." Hanna, who had breast augmentation and
rhinoplasty, refused to do surgeries that involve fat removal. "No, I
won't do any tummy tucks, liposuction," she said. When asked why,
she responded, "Because I find, like, it's easy, and it's a discipline to
actually to lose the weight and to work out. It's really easy to lose
weight. It's just, work off more than eat. It's a very easy concept."
Casey also believes surgery is not needed to sculpt the abdomen: "I'm
a forty-year-old woman who's going through middle-age spread. I
work out a lot. If I would just quit drinking a bottle of wine every
night, I'm pretty sure my belly would go away. These are things that
I can fix on my own if I'm motivated enough. You can suck in your
gut, but you can't suck in your breasts." She was fine with having
bilateral breast reduction (which came with "free" liposuction in
her armpits that her surgeon "threw in") but not liposuction in her
abdominal area. In her view, dietary changes—particularly laying
off the alcohol—would suffice. Jenna, Hanna, and Casey's perspective is consistent with cultural beliefs that behavioral efforts alone
are sufficient to achieve weight loss and a firm, sculpted body. Of
course, participants who struggled to change their body shape and
size would vehemently contest this claim, illustrating how notions of
bodily control are shaped by a participant's ideologies and personal
body-modification struggles.

Participants blamed a host of factors for making their body parts
difficult to sculpt. Hormonal changes that come with menopause,
they bemoaned, irreversibly changed their bodies. Pregnancy and
breastfeeding were frequently mentioned culprits that left women

with stomachs stretched and breasts "ruined," "shriveled," and looking like "raisin boobs." They also blamed aging and gravity for sagging breasts. Jasmine even intimated that she had a psychological disorder that resulted in a pathological relationship to food. She pointed out that, since the age of five, she had struggled with her relationship to food and stated that inside her mind "something's not wired correctly." Of course, participants emphasized that they simply could not help being born with a certain face or body shape. All these factors led them to conclude that surgery was "needed."

Ultimately, this reasoning allows women to account for cosmetic surgery. Within a self-improvement culture, women package cosmetic surgery as a reasonable, necessary, and responsible act. They have little choice but to have surgery because some factor beyond their control (e.g., biology, gravity, a disorder) constrained the amount of visible change possible without surgical intervention. Before turning to surgery, they gave their best efforts using socially acceptable means such as dieting and exercising. This reasoning allows them to symbolically justify their decisions and distance themselves from unnecessary surgery—surgery that involves body parts that can be manipulated without the surgeon's knife or surgery undertaken without first making concerted efforts at change.

Good Surgeries

Participants' boundary work also involved differentiating their good, acceptable, and "necessary" surgeries from bad and unacceptable ones. In their view, the former are done by competent surgeons and do not involve psychological pathology or unrealistic expectations. They also draw on self-improvement rhetoric. Moreover, they are done for oneself, not others. Finally, good and acceptable surgeries have admirable motives and allow participants to still look like themselves and retain a sense of self—especially a modest self that is not preoccupied with sexuality.

Hiring Competent Surgeons

During their interviews, participants discussed how they picked their surgeons. Several participants stressed that they paid for what they believed was the best surgeon in their area. Janet (who spent $30,000 on face-lifts, a breast augmentation, and a tummy tuck) and Lacy (whose parents spent an estimated $20,000 on her liposuction) went so far as to say that if one cannot afford the best surgeon, then one should not have surgery at all. For Janet, going to a bad surgeon was the equivalent of buying a used car that has been in an accident. The "results will be unhappy." She continued, "It's never going to be like a new car. You're going to save money but you're going to end up spending more money because it's inferior." Paying more meant she was not going to a "hack in Brazil," to borrow Casey's words. She saw the higher price tag as a way of minimizing risk, explaining that surgery was not the place to penny-pinch. Pricier surgeons, in these participants' view, were well worth their fees. Kerrie said, "I didn't want to bargain when it came to my body."[5]

Although a high price tag signified surgeon competency for a few, participants generally exhibited budget consciousness. They did not merely find the most expensive surgeon and then come up with a way to pay. For them, good surgeries meant hiring surgeons they thought were competent but could also afford without accruing an unreasonable amount of debt. Participants who borrowed money or financed their procedures were keen to share that they had either paid off these debts or were making steady progress toward doing so. In this way, they framed surgery as a responsible financial decision, not a reckless one. In our sample, there were a few exceptions. We discuss Rebecca's story later in this chapter and Ana Marie's story in the next.

Along with price, participants turned to other cues to determine surgeon competency. They began with the internet. For example, using the Google search engine, Grace typed in the procedure, along with the city and state where she lives. Of course, a surgeon's place on a search engine results list was not the only factor she used, but it did matter to her. She explained, "If you Google 'breast augmentation' [in my city and state], he's the first one. He has his own billboard here. He's just top ranked. He's five out of five stars. He has a lot of awards, a lot of recognition." So while she initially relied on search engine results, she needed more evidence, noting the surgeon's marketing presence and awards. Another frequently mentioned tool was a surgeon's online portfolio. Participants perused surgeons' before and after photos to assess whether their work appeared "unnatural" or "fake." These photos helped them evaluate a surgeon's ability to achieve the natural fake that the vast majority of them coveted.

Certification and training, particularly in the United States, was also important to participants. Jessica, who had breast augmentation in the 1970s, described her surgeon as a "trailblazer." In her understanding, he was one of only three surgeons in the United States who was "fully [board] certified" at the time. In their minds, knowing a surgeon was certified reduced the fear that something might go wrong during surgery. Ashley said, "I knew there were risks but I wasn't afraid of the risks [of having breast augmentation] because I knew I was going to a board-certified plastic surgeon and the work was being done in the United States. Everything was clean." Linda stated frankly that she was comfortable having her cosmetic procedures (including nonsurgical procedures) only if a doctor who had completed medical school and residency with a focus on plastic surgery performed them. She voiced skepticism regarding professionals who completed specialized training in one- or two-day seminars. Casey too emphasized how her surgery was not "back alley creepy" and was performed in a university hospital.

Even the four participants who had surgery abroad (largely to reduce costs) insisted that they hired safe and qualified surgeons whom they vetted. All four were culturally connected to the countries where they had surgery; these countries were thus not "foreign" to them. For example, Parvina, whose family is from Iran, had rhinoplasty there. In her view, "Iran is number one in plastic surgery, noses, and everything." She believed she "was in better hands there than [she] would have been here" and underscored that her surgeon was educated in Belgium. She referred affectionately to him as "twinkle hands" because she thought he was so skilled at creating noses that "looked so natural."[6] Similarly, Elaina had rhinoplasty and ear surgery in her birth country of Mexico. She warned others, "You just have to do your research first before you go. You don't just go with Joe Blow." Sylvia and Taylor also had ties to the countries where they had surgery. Sylvia went with a surgeon (in Mexico) with whom a family member had a positive experience, and Taylor had surgery (in Colombia) done by a surgeon whom a family member worked for as a nurse.

Although our focus here is on recurrent cues participants used to discern a competent surgeon, two participants mentioned the influence of surgeons' personal status characteristics. While these characteristics surfaced organically in only two interviews, we nevertheless mention them because they illustrate the importance of status characteristics such as gender, age, race, ethnicity, and physical appearance.[7] First is Kristen, who intentionally sought an older male Asian surgeon. Kristen is black and twenty-four years of age. She expressed disapproval of a family friend who went to a female surgeon:

> I think . . . women . . . have preconceived notions in our minds. I think, as a man, he just respects your decision more. I just didn't want a female doctor. I wanted a male doctor. I wanted him to be kind of older, so he's been doing it awhile. . . . Call me prejudiced, but I wanted Asian because, just like when [they] do my nails, they're really detail oriented.

Her choice to go with a male surgeon is consistent with the rest of the women in our sample—the large majority of whom hired a male surgeon. This is likely a function of availability because women are underrepresented in this medical specialty.[8] However, her preference for a male surgeon runs contrary to research showing that most female patients considering cosmetic surgery do not have a sex preference. And of those who do, research suggests that nearly all prefer a woman.[9] Kristen's belief that Asian doctors are more detail oriented reflects scholarship on the beauty service work industry that documents clients' widespread racial biases and stereotypes.[10] It may also be driven by the model minority stereotype of Asians collectively having a strong work ethic[11]—a stereotype reinforced in part by narrow media depictions.[12]

Unlike Kristen, who prioritized gender, age, and race, Martha, age sixty-seven, focused on physical appearance. She considered five surgeons for her face-lift. She nixed one because of bad reviews. However, she rejected the others because of the way they looked. One had dilated eyes, which "spooked her." "A couple of them looked kind of creepy. They had been overdone." And one, "very obviously, had plastic surgery himself." Martha was clearly uncomfortable with the physical appearance of these surgeons, even crossing some off her list because they appeared to have had cosmetic surgery. There is, undeniably, an irony in criticizing a plastic surgeon for having had cosmetic surgery when one is looking to do the same. Yet Martha's perspective calls attention to the overwhelming preference for the natural fake both for herself and in others. If a surgeon had work done, Martha preferred that it not *look* as if they had.

Some participants' statements that emphasized the necessity of paying for the "best" surgeons thus exhibited classist undertones. Furthermore, while likely not intentionally racist, participants passed ethnocentric judgment not only on women who hire surgeons outside the United States but also on the surgeons themselves and the medical context in which they practice. When she says she did not go to "a hack in Brazil," Casey reinforces a negative stereotype of medicine in the global south, real or not, as having subpar medical standards. She not only condemns the imaginary irresponsible woman who travels south to save a buck but denigrates the surgeons there and the medical culture in which they practice. In participants' minds, safe cosmetic surgery allegedly takes place in the United States by a presumably white or Asian surgeon. This surgeon has trained at an American institution of higher learning or someplace comparable. They envision a pristine office with soft lighting, orchids, and furniture with clean lines and a modern feel. (As Lacy said, she selected a surgeon who had a "clean *modern* waiting room.") In contrast, cosmetic surgery in the global south purportedly is done by unregulated practitioners, at times not even in a clinic or a hospital. As Ana Marie commented, "bad stuff" *can* happen when one has cosmetic surgery abroad "because the penalties are not as harsh as here [in the United States]."

Being Psychologically Sound and Not Exhibiting Pathology

Participants also had firm beliefs about who should or should not have cosmetic surgery. Like themselves, surgery candidates should be emotionally stable and psychologically sound. In contrast is the anonymous surgical other, whom participants associate with pathology.[13] In their opinion, people who exhibit extreme insecurity, self-hatred, or a mental disorder are not appropriate surgery candidates.

When asked whether she would recommend cosmetic surgery to others, Lorna said:

> I would recommend it. I would totally recommend it, because my life is better. I don't have any reservations. If people want to have cosmetic surgery, more power to you. Go, you, . . . if you can and it makes you feel better. Now if you have other, deeper psychological issues, like you're an alcoholic and you're doing this, you're just trying to fill a void, [then] that's a different issue. But if you want to go get a tummy tuck because you know you're hot stuff and you want to walk around on the beach, then go do it! And I think that's where mine comes from.

For Lorna, those with "deeper psychological issues" should not turn to surgery to compensate for their psychological inadequacies. Instead, she described a surgery candidate whose confidence is already high and who uses surgery to enhance this confidence. Lorna was particularly outspoken and gregarious. She oozed self-assurance and exhibited wit. She is an elementary school music teacher who described herself as a performer and proclaimed, "I love to sing! I love to smile! I love to act!" In our hour-plus interview, she used *confident* (or its variant) about a dozen times and said that cosmetic surgery had further increased her confidence and outgoing personality. Others, she believes, should use cosmetic surgery only the way she did: as valued added to an already rich life.

Similarly, Jasmine stressed that she was in a good mental state before surgery. Before having breast augmentation, a full body lift, and liposuction at age twenty-three, she talked to her sister at length. Their conversation centered on her psychological constitution. She explained:

> I wanted to make sure I was happy with me and okay with me—[that I] like me—before doing it and go, I'm not doing this because I'm unhappy with myself. I'm doing this because this is uncomfortable or I'd prefer it to be this way, not because I hate everything and my life would be fixed. . . . I didn't want to be in a place where I thought that that would fix my life. I

> wanted to be fine with my life and want to enhance it, because I felt like if I did it to fix something—like fix my life—then that's what it would hinge on. And if my life wasn't fixed, then I would not—I would hate it. I would regret the decision. So I'm like, okay, I'm good, I'm me, I'm awesome, but this is uncomfortable, so I think I'm going to do this to help not be so uncomfortable.

Although she was "uncomfortable" in her body, Jasmine insisted that she did not use cosmetic surgery to fix her life. She was in touch with herself enough to know that this would be futile. Kali too emphasized how surgery is not for those who have deep emotional issues: "If it's just the physical part of it that's making you unhappy and you want the cosmetic surgery, go ahead and do it. If it's something deeper, then you need to figure that out." Participants thus stressed that they did not use surgery to resolve serious psychological or emotional problems. And they frowned on those who do, advising that they should resolve these problems before going under the knife.

According to participants, emotionally stable patients also do not abuse surgery or become addicted. They admonished celebrities who "overdid it." Parvina's description of people who do not know when to stop was particularly scathing: "You're going drastic. Like, Heidi Montag had seventeen surgeries in one day. That's retarded!" Hazel too had strong opinions on this matter: "I mean, there are people who are addicted to plastic surgery. You hear about somebody having eleven procedures in one day. Something's not right up here. I mean, that's insane. I wouldn't even get my breasts and my nose done at the same time!" By emphatically rebuking "addicts" and impugning the mental stability of these allegedly pathological surgical others, participants demonstrated their own sound mind and reasonable comportment. Martha's words capture an expression we heard repeatedly, an expression that explicitly denigrates the surgical other by saying one is not like this other: "I'm not a plastic surgery junkie!"

Participants distinguished themselves from addicts who overdo surgery, but one participant openly shared her struggles with repeat surgeries. At the time we met Rebecca, she was forty and divorced. As a teen, her Southern California schoolmates made fun of her. She admitted to having low body esteem. When her friend had cosmetic surgery resulting in a nose she found "small and cute," Rebecca followed suit. She had never felt pretty and hoped surgery would help: "Oh, maybe this will make me pretty. Just make me pretty and people won't think I'm ugly anymore." Surgery at age nineteen did in fact change how she saw herself, but only for a brief period.

Around age twenty-two, Rebecca started disliking her nose again. She was not certain if it was "the scar tissue or what," but she "saw pictures [of herself] and didn't like it." She thought her nose was "crooked [and] a mess." She turned to a surgeon a friend recommended. The second surgery was disappointing. Unhappy with these results, she did another, then another, followed by yet another.[14] After one of these many surgeries, her body rejected a surgical implant, resulting in repeated infections. She made multiple attempts to get rid of the scar tissue these surgeries left behind. In her words: "Laser. Laser. Laser." Two decades after her first surgery, she lamented that she still has "massive scarring," for which she continues to have laser treatments.

Despite the failure of her nose surgeries, Rebecca had breast augmentation at age twenty-four. She explained that it was partly because she had a line of credit available and partly because she was emotionally confused at the time: "You go through a divorce, you get a little cuckoo, and you just want to do a bunch of stuff to be different." She admitted that during the divorce she lost quite a bit of weight and suffered from anorexia nervosa.

In stark contrast to Lorna, an aura of despair surrounds Rebecca. Cosmetic surgery, she said, has regretfully consumed her life. She confessed to being financially unstable, explaining that repeat surgeries have drained her bank accounts. She is self-employed, selling items on eBay: "Now I'm broke. I can't even work because now I can't go to work. I'm having [laser] treatments all the time. Seriously. It's embarrassing. It's humiliating. It's awful." When reflecting on her experiences with cosmetic surgery, she said with a sigh of exasperation and tentativeness, "I guess I'm just glad to be done with it, but it depresses me. It depresses me that I wasted my whole life, and it was just so stupid. I'm really just angry at myself. I'm angry that I didn't realize that I was going to a doctor that was just messing with me. He obviously didn't know what he was doing. I look back and I'm like, 'God, I was so stupid.' I have a lot of regrets. A lot of regrets."

Rebecca blames herself as well as her surgeon. She was never satisfied with the appearance of her nose, but this was in part because her surgeon was not able to deliver the results she desired. At age forty, she concludes that she wasted her life because she spent extensive time, money, and physical and emotional energy on cosmetic surgery. She was passionate that others should not have surgery, citing it as an "evil" that she "wished was never invented." She continued, "It's become out of hand these days."

Despite saying she is done with cosmetic surgery, Rebecca told us that if financial means permitted, she would redo her breasts. With age, they have lowered, and she wants "them more perky and more filled out, more lifted." She is also contemplating a tummy tuck. At the time of our interview, a clinical trial in California (likely the same one Kali participated in) was offering to pay women to have abdominoplasty. Rebecca intended to reach out to the researchers after our meeting. When asked, "Do you feel you can stop [having surgeries]?," she replied, "Maybe not. It's around me, too. You know what I mean? It's there, it's there, it's there. This person's getting this done. This person's getting that done. It's almost like you have to keep up. Yeah, maybe I can't stop." Her financial situation, psychological struggles, and her inability to stop having cosmetic surgery reflect characteristics of the surgical other from which so many participants worked to distance themselves.

Having Realistic Expectations

Our participants are not cultural dupes. As Chapter 2 highlights, they are aware that women's beauty ideals are fabrications that involve Photoshopping and other technological tricks. They know that only a lucky few innately embody these ideals. Consistent with this cultural savvy and the belief that surgery is for the psychologically sound, they also believe that good surgery begins with reasonable expectations. Typically, they articulated this in terms of the absence of perfection. For example, Darla said, "I paid a lot of money, [but] I'm not looking for 100 percent perfection." Casey too showed no desire for perfection: "Nobody's perfect in my opinion. I don't feel like you have to reach perfection." And when asked what she hoped surgery would accomplish, Linda replied, "Having softer features, looking less tired, looking a tiny bit better, but trying to have very realistic expectations." This realistic attitude was also evident *after* surgery, as Kali's postoperative comments reveal: "I'm pleased with the results, I wouldn't mind if they were better, but I understand that these were the realistic expectations." When Penelope's eyelid surgery left her with a visible scar above her left eye, she said it did not bother her and remarked, "It comes with the territory."

Research shows that surgeons evaluate patient expectations and prefer patients who exhibit reasonableness.[15] In our interviews, participants disclosed that their surgeons practiced this type of vetting. Grace's surgeon asked about her motives "because he wanted to make sure that I had a reasonable mind-set about my own goals. Because anyone going in there expecting perfection, that doctor is going to shoot them down." Janet's surgeon vets his clients in the same manner: "You see, Dr. ——, he will not even operate on you if he thinks you have any mental problems whatsoever. . . . If he thinks that your expectations are not what you're going to get, he refuses to work." This type of vetting is part of a larger package of patient interactions that help surgeons convey professionalism and distinguish themselves from quacks. It is one strategy used to minimize the stigma that surrounds the profession. Thus, surgeons and patients alike do boundary work by taking the moral high ground. From patients' vantage point, they are reasonable (unlike, say, patients who demand perfection). From surgeons' vantage point, they are professionally responsible (unlike, say, surgeons who perform surgery on anyone in the name of the almighty dollar).

Having Surgery for Me, Me, Me!

Self-improvement discourses are one side of the cosmetic surgery paradox. A makeover and self-help culture encourages women to work on themselves using a plethora of products and services. Whether it is striving to obtain more education, to get a promotion at work, or to look and feel better, women are encouraged to be their best. This is purportedly "because you're worth it," something L'Oréal has been telling women since the 1970s.[16] Given this cultural rhetoric of bettering oneself, it is not surprising that participants framed cosmetic surgery as an empowering choice.[17] Moreover, it is a choice done for oneself, sometimes even as a gift to oneself. (For example, Marianne's surgery was a birthday gift to herself, and Lavanna's was a Christmas gift to herself). Allison, who beams with confidence, exemplifies this for-the-self perspective. She does not shy from it, stating, "It wasn't for a man. . . . It wasn't for anybody else. . . . It's all about me. It's always me. Me, me, me!"

Surgery for "me, me, me" unequivocally means *not* for significant others. Participants made this point clear. For example, at the time of her breast surgery, Carla borrowed money from her boyfriend (whom she later married) and the father of her three children. She was disappointed with the look, size, and feel of her breasts after breastfeeding her children. She said others joked that her breasts were his: "Sometimes people like to say, 'Oh, they're his, 'cause he paid for it.' And I'm like, 'No!' Because . . . I paid him back. I did this for myself, and I did not do this for anybody." When asked if she takes offense when others say this, she replied with an emphatic, "Yes!" She continued to insist that surgery was done for herself: "I felt like I don't want it to be connected to anybody but myself because I didn't like the way I looked. It wasn't what anybody else told me. It was what I felt." Jessica too was quick to convey that she did not have breast augmentation for her boyfriend. She said, "He's not a breast man. He didn't see any point in [the surgery]."

Accompanying this for-the-self rhetoric is criticism of women who did not have surgery for themselves. "A single woman thinks it's going to help her find a husband. That's the wrong reason to do it," quipped Heather—a resounding indictment of women like Caitlin who explicitly use surgery to obtain a partner. Linda said that if one tries to have surgery for someone else, it is a failed strategy: "If you're trying to impress someone or you're trying to keep up with the Joneses, that never really works. . . . You can only be your best self." Markedly, she emphasizes the one thing she feels she can control— her ability to be her best self. Similarly, Sylvia condemned her friend who had surgery to fit in: "I know somebody . . . doing it because they're around these beautiful women that have this perfect body. I've seen it myself, and I feel bad for that person because they're not doing it for themselves. They're doing it to fit in."

Having Good Motives

Psychological and Emotional Well-Being

According to participants, acceptable surgeries have commendable motives. Good motives center on improving psychological and physical well-being. In contrast, bad motives center on women's sexuality. As reported in Chapter 2, feeling that they do not live up to cultural standards of femininity, participants turn to the tools at their disposal, including cosmetic surgery. This is seen as an acceptable motive. To be sure, participants construct an image of a smart, competent, and psychologically sound woman who uses modern technology to improve herself. For example, during her interview, Allison, now fifty, mentioned several times that she is "okay" with her body. She said that her life philosophy included a simple tenet: If she could improve something about her body, she would certainly try. She discussed where she believed this outlook stemmed from:

> I was brought up by a single mom who was very comfortable [with herself]. She had a boob job, but she did it to fix [them]. They were a mess. They just looked horrible, and she wanted them to look better. And I was brought up by two very strong women who were very comfortable with who they were, and I think I learned from them. And what we have is what we have, and if we can fix it, let's fix it. And if not, we'll move on, but we're okay with all of this.

An upbringing with strong female role models meant Allison was not hung up on body issues. If she could improve her body, fine. If she could not, then life would be okay. In Allison's case, she was unhappy with her breasts. So at age thirty-two, she had them done. She was able to "fix it"—the technology was there, and she had the means to pay for surgery.

Over and over again, participants said that cosmetic surgery is a technological tool women *should* take advantage of. And although they admitted that this type of surgery comes with risks, they said "science" has made cosmetic surgery relatively safe, especially if one heeds doctor's orders. The vast majority of participants held the opinion that cosmetic surgery is "modern" and "safe" and explained that they were just taking advantage of these modern technologies to better themselves. From their perspective, increasing body satisfaction, self-esteem, and confidence, as well as comfort with and in one's body, are all praiseworthy motives. For example, Janet said, "It lets you change what you want to change [and] become more confident." Casey said, "I'm really glad that I did it. I'm more comfortable. . . . [I] have better self-image. It wasn't a huge life changer. It's not like I was reborn or anything." In fact, all the women we spoke with invoked psychological well-being in some form. Cosmetic surgery made them more comfortable with their bodies, which in turn, brought greater confidence and self-esteem. It was not necessarily a "huge life changer" as Casey put it, but it certainly helped boost psychological and emotional well-being.

Physical Well-Being
A few participants also cited self-improvement in the name of physical health. For example, when discussing her motivations for liposuction, Nadine mentioned that "it's not healthy to have belly fat." While Nadine reasons that the removal of fat automatically *creates* a healthier body, Lacy used surgery as an incentive to *maintain* a healthy body. Because her parents paid a large sum of money for her liposuction, surgery motivated her to lead a healthy lifestyle. Lacy admitted she would feel shame going back to her surgeon if she did not retain her new physique:

> There are probably people that have gotten liposuction and gone right back to the way they were. For me, that doesn't make any sense. Because my parents paid all this money and I went through all of this recovery—so to have to go back there, and then, you know, I'd feel kinda, you know, embarrassed if I had to go back to my plastic surgeon and I was like, hey, so remember all that work you did? Well, I know how you told me I shouldn't do this, but I did.

Surgery prompted concerted efforts to work out and eat better. She felt she became more aware of her body after surgery. She became a vegan (switching from vegetarianism, which she had been practicing for several years). Pilates, yoga, and walking were now aspects of her daily life. Just as researchers have found that weight loss surgery can serve as a point of rebirth,[18] participants used liposuction or abdominoplasty as a lifestyle reboot. After ongoing efforts at weight loss and body sculpting that led to limited success, surgery served as the final turning point. In Susan's words, "But now, I think I take better care of myself, and I have to maintain, so that I don't get back to that point." Kristen said it has made her appreciate her body more. "[I take] care of my body more. . . . I just appreciate myself. I love myself more." Or as Taylor reflected, "I felt like I needed to do this in order to push myself to be healthier, to keep up with it. I felt like, before, I would try different things and lose weight and gain it right back. I felt like if I did this, I would have more of an investment into myself, keeping up with my weight and eating healthier, just changing my whole lifestyle."

The importance of participants' self-improvement language cannot be overstated. It mirrors larger cultural discourses that praise women for embarking on body projects. Participants said that having cosmetic surgery was no different from "putting on makeup," "going to the gym," or "seeing a therapist." These are all ways women *can* improve themselves and are *expected* to improve themselves. In fact, Kali felt that women who have cosmetic surgery are more self-aware than women who do not. This is because they are taking control of something they are not happy about. As she put it, "I don't even think it's fake. I think it's more in touch with yourself than someone who doesn't get a cosmetic surgery because they're aware that something isn't what they want it to be. They're taking a step."

Preserving an Authentic and Unique Self

A final form of boundary work emerged in our conversations with participants. This form of boundary work allowed participants to distinguish themselves from surgical others, justify their surgeries, and reaffirm a certain sense of self. According to participants, good surgeries do not involve a loss of self, while bad surgeries lead patients to look in the mirror and ask, to use Lavanna's words, "Who is this?" So although cosmetic surgery involves altering physical appearance, participants stressed that they are still the "same person." Still being this same person—their *authentic* self—is likely why, when asked what life would have been like without surgery, the majority said it was not a game changer. They insisted they were still themselves—just version 2.0: enhanced, improved, better. It is also likely why surgery is about normalcy. Despite surgery, they are still mothers, daughters, sisters, workers, and students who go about their everyday activities, only with a little more confidence. Finally, this exaltation of an authentic self is likely why participants are critical of results that are extreme, obvious, and do not appear natural. The inconspicuous natural fake enables them to avoid dramatically altering their appearance and, by extension, who they are. This is especially because, for women, appearance and the self are very much intertwined. Despite cosmetic surgery, they remain true to themselves.

Being the same person after surgery, above all, involves not altering the body in a way that makes one unrecognizable. Lavanna's perspective on celebrities who "go overboard" illuminates this point. In her view, Kim Kardashian has undergone so much change under the knife that she does not look like the same person. Such radical changes are "spooky," "scary," and "alien"—terms she and other participants used. She is equally critical of Nicki Minaj: "She looks like some things are not real on her body. . . . It's not real looking!" For this reason, Lavanna places limits on the type of cosmetic surgery she is willing to have. "So I don't think I'll alter my face. I still need to look like the same person," she remarked. While she is open to having a future face-lift that pulls her face back, she disses chin and cheek implants. These implants, she believes, would dramatically alter her appearance. Maintaining her defining facial characteristics is crucial for Lavanna. It allows her to retain her authentic self and avoid an identity crisis. As she told us, "If you look in the mirror and you don't look like the same person to you, that's scary. I don't ever want to look in the mirror and I'm like, 'Who is this?' No." In the same way, Parvina commented on those who, famous or not, overdo surgery: "You're like, what the hell did they do to themselves? They don't even look human anymore." In her boundary work, Parvina distances herself from these unnamed others who she believes have gone too far. Going too far means one does not look human, let alone like oneself.

Reese's criticism of the now-canceled reality television show *The Swan* provides further evidence of participants' view that surgery should not make one unrecognizable. The Fox network series aired extreme makeovers that involved cosmetic surgery. The audience witnessed a candidate's dramatic physical transformation with results that, at times, rendered her unrecognizable to loved ones. Reese cringed when discussing the show: "*The Swan* thing just creeps me out. Somebody goes somewhere looking one way and then comes back . . . not even recognizable. Like, I just, ugh, ugh, ugh [*shudders*]. I would feel like an alien in my own body if I did something to my face, I think." Like Lavanna, Reese is cautious about having work done on her face because manipulating the face opens the door to feeling "alien" in one's own body.

This concern for retaining an authentic self might also be why our four participants who had face-lifts—Janet, Marianne, Martha, and Penelope—said they did not "look drawn" or have a forever "wind blown" or "surprised look." Instead, they insisted they still looked "like me." In fact, Martha said that she had a moment of panic weeks following her face-lift. Even after most of the bruising and swelling had subsided, she was struggling to recognize herself: "It was kind of creepy because I didn't even look remotely like myself. It kind of scared me." Her friends and family members agreed, which elevated her anxiety. Thankfully, after a few months she was able to say with much relief: "I look like me now." While it is impossible to know if she truly started looking more like her former self as the healing progressed or whether she adjusted to a new normal, the point remains, she was relieved when she came to believe that she looked like herself again.

This concern for retaining one's self is also perhaps why some participants were leery about Botox. Although quite a few participants had used, were using, or were open to Botox use in the future, a handful were apprehensive that Botox might create an unnatural or alien-like look. For example, Allison was open to different cosmetic procedures. But she drew the line with Botox: "No Botox. I make fun of people, I'm sorry to say. I'm bad about that. I cannot stand it when somebody smiles and they don't look like they're smiling or they look alien to me. . . . There's something very bizarre about that look. It's not natural." In her view, Botox injections, just like bad face-lifts, are "not natural" and make a woman unrecognizable, potentially resulting in alienation and a loss of self.

When discussing the importance of an authentic true-to-themselves postoperative self, participants simultaneously emphasized retaining a unique self. Several participants made this point by invoking anti-Barbie sentiments. Specifically, they did not want to exit surgery looking like the iconic American fashion doll. So while Barbie may be a feminine beauty icon, she is also a cultural placeholder for the generic. Consequently, if a woman looks like Barbie, then she looks neither like herself nor unique. Despite using cosmetic surgery to embody cultural norms of femininity—norms that are inherently standardized—participants still paradoxically hoped to be one of a kind.

For example, Marianne joked that she wanted to come out of surgery looking like herself, just her younger self: "But I mean, I think people look good that don't look like everybody else. See, to me, the vanilla Barbies are no longer attractive. I've become desensitized to the look—I don't want to look like that. [After surgery] I still want to look like me, just a younger version of me [*laughs*]." Marianne pairs vanilla with Barbie to describe an image of something she does not want to embody—the prosaic, common, everyday. As reported in Chapter 2, her affluent social networks were influential in her decision to have cosmetic surgery. Being embedded in these circles in Dallas desensitized her to breast implants. The Barbie look was so common that she felt it was not attractive, and it was one of the reasons she "only got 135CC [implants, or about a one-cup-size increase], whereas a lot of women are getting 300s and 600s [about a two- to four-cup-size increase]."[19] This was Marianne's way of distinguishing herself from the vanilla Barbies around her.

Similarly, Penelope emphasized that she is not Barbie: "I think I have a distinct look that's different and that it stands out. And that's what I think is beautiful. That you're kind of different, you're not a carbon copy. I'm certainly not a Barbie doll." Looking like Barbie is undesirable because it means looking like a "carbon copy" or having a "cookie-cutter look." In sum, participants denigrated surgical others (including movie and reality television stars) for losing themselves in the process of having cosmetic surgery. By making dramatic and obvious physical changes, they compromised their authentic selves. In contrast, good surgery makes possible the retention of an authentic and uniquely beautiful self.

The Moral and Modest Self

But who is this authentic and unique self? The following exchange with Taylor hints at the answer. It also shows various forms of boundary work. She recalled a conversation with a few friends before surgery:

> TAYLOR: Some of my friends, when I mentioned that I was having the surgery, they were like, "No, don't do that. You're going to be one of *those* girls."
> INTERVIEWER: What do you mean, one of *those* girls?
> TAYLOR: Just, you know, constantly going in to get procedures. You know, boob jobs, nose jobs, lip injections, whatever else they do. It wasn't until I explained to them I'm not trying to do this to be a Barbie doll. I just want to get a little figure that I've been trying to get at the gym, and it just doesn't work.

Unable to sculpt her body at the gym, thereby making surgery "necessary," Taylor had surgery to obtain a hallmark of femininity—a "little figure." She then explicitly distances herself from the surgical other. She points out that she does not want to be a generic Barbie doll and reassures her friends that she will not become "one of *those* girls." Her tone is derogatory when she clarifies that *those* girls are having multiple surgeries—"boob jobs, nose jobs, lip injections, whatever."

Taylor's concern with not becoming "one of *those* girls" is loaded with moral undercurrents. Boundary work separates participants from surgical others not just in terms of the types of surgery and the circumstances under which they take place. Importantly, it also creates moral boundaries. The authentic self that participants hope to retain despite surgery is a moral self. Even if cosmetic surgery is done in the name of beauty, unlike for *those* girls, for our participants it is not an obsession. Participants see the pursuit of psychological, emotional, and physical health as good motivation. Beauty obsession is not.

The voices of other participants shed further light on this authentic self while showing the centrality of morality and modesty. Although surgery allows participants to feel feminine and more confident in their bodies, including their sexuality, they went out of their way to say that they are not women who are preoccupied with or who prioritize sexuality. For example, Jessica said, "It really didn't have anything to do with sexuality as much as the ideal woman." Kerrie said, "I didn't want to be out there like a Playboy model or anything. I just really did it for myself." Heather stated, "I mean, you have to be happy with yourself and other things too. You can't just be all boobs. . . . I'd be horrified if that was me." And Grace explained, "I would say just to try to keep it natural because you don't want that to become who you are. You don't want people to notice your boobs before they notice your eyes."

Grace insists that she is more than her altered body part. Others should notice her eyes first—the metaphorical entrance to her soul. They should notice her—her entire being—not only her augmented breasts. She emphasizes how the natural fake helps people see her and not just her "boobs," ostensibly because natural-appearing results are discreet. These quotes also reinforce other recurring themes—surgery for self, internal happiness, and ideal femininity—while simultaneously downplaying sexuality. Kerrie is not "a Playboy model." Heather is steadfastly not "all boobs."

Participants who had breast surgery were particularly keen to downplay their sexuality. They did this by dressing more conservatively after surgery. Vanessa, a twenty-seven-year-old single mom, said she was flattered by the attention she received after surgery. At the same time she was concerned that men were attracted to her breasts and not her: "Because I know the attention that I get now, it's because of them." She continued, "I think that's probably why I cover up more, because then you really cannot tell. Yeah. That's why I wear a lot of loose blouses. . . . During the day, I'm very covered up, especially when I have my daughter." Vanessa insists that others cannot tell she had surgery—thanks to the natural fake—and that she is not flaunting her breasts. She is mindful of dressing conservatively when she is with her daughter. A good mom, she implies, does not wantonly display her sexuality. Similarly, Sarah, who is thirty-eight and engaged, does not want to draw attention to her breasts. After surgery, she changed her clothing style: "I started to choose clothing that wasn't so—I had always worn very tailored outfits before, and I wasn't interested in wearing things that were as formfitting. I didn't want to because I knew that the size of my chest had changed. . . . I didn't want to draw attention to the girls." Dressing modestly is no doubt a strategy consistent with passing as surgically unaltered.

College student Kaylee shared a story about an experience in her Psychology of Women course that further illustrates how participants do not want to be defined by their surgery or be seen as women who prioritize sex. During one class students started relating breast implants to porn and sex. Kaylee wanted to "stand up and be like, 'Do I look like a porn star to you?'" However, assessing that she was outnumbered and that it was not a safe space in which to retort, she remained quiet. She continued to take class notes. During our interview, however, she vented. She insisted she is not about "flaunting it or showing it off":

> Some people, I'm scared they'll just be immediate to judge and be like, "You did this for someone else" or "You did this to be more attractive." I haven't been sexually active in years. I haven't dated in years. I didn't do it so I could date again. I wanted to do this for me. Like I mentioned before, people may have a different [view] of cosmetic surgery, especially breast implants, because usually women do it to show off or something.

Kaylee defends her moral self. She is not the hypersexualized stereotypical woman who obtains breasts implants to "show off." While others may associate breast augmentation with sex and sexuality, this is not an accurate depiction of her. Similarly, Leanne, who lives in Southern California, insisted she is not a "beach bunny" or a "river rat." When asked to clarify the term *river rat*, she replied:

> When I say "river rat," I mean all those, the women that go hang out on the boats at the river, and you know, they're drunk and [in] teeny-tiny tops and their boobs are everywhere, and

that is who they are. And that was not who I was. And that's
not what I wanted to be. I think that's who they are. I think
that's their identity. And for me doing it, it was more, you
know, self-esteem.

In the same breath that Leanne invokes a noble motivation—psychological health—she disparages the "river rats" who exhibit lasciviousness
and insobriety. It is "their identity"—most certainly not hers.

Boundary Work as Identity Work

Participants' accounts of their surgeries exhibit a distancing from
surgical others who do not exemplify praiseworthy attributes. In their
opinion, their surgeries, which embody the natural fake, are necessary in the context of a makeover culture. They paid good money and
turned to reputable, recommended, well-rated, well-educated, and
well-trained surgeons. As patients, they had reasonable expectations
about what surgery could achieve, and they did not use surgery to
address serious psychological shortcomings. Moreover, surgery was
done for themselves in the name of self-improvement—not for a significant other or to keep up with peers. All these accounts allow them
to turn the cosmetic surgery paradox on its head by showing that
cosmetic surgery is a justifiable and even necessary solution to cultural pressures. Furthermore, they show that the stigma of cosmetic
surgery does not apply to them. Their surgeries are reasonable, responsible, and justified. The stigma of cosmetic surgery applies only
to other patients and other types of surgery that are not performed
under these reasonable, responsible, and justified circumstances.

Boundary work is a form of identity work. Identity work is the
activities people engage in that allow them to create, present, and
sustain a personal identity congruent with their self-concept.[20] Participants construct boundaries, including moral boundaries, that so-
lidify and project a desired sense of self. While cosmetic surgery may
have altered their physical appearance, participants professed that
surgery did not constitute their entire being. They denigrated others
for losing themselves in the process of having cosmetic surgery. By
making dramatic and obvious physical changes, these surgical oth-

ers compromise their authentic self. In contrast, participants after surgery are still their same recognizable and unique selves.

This unique self, they insisted, is a moral self that is sexually modest. Because cosmetic surgery is about body aesthetics, like the students in Kaylee's college classroom, people associate cosmetic surgery with women's sexuality. Women who have cosmetic surgery are aware of this stereotype and actively resist it. Breasts, in particular, are sexual signifiers in our society.[21] Thus, participants who had breast augmentation were especially concerned that others would view them as hypersexual. Yes, they underwent breast surgery, but this does not mean that they are preoccupied with sex. Boundary work means reframing and claiming—I am this, and I am adamantly not that. In this case, reframing involves the assertion that good surgeries are done by moral women who are trying only to improve their lives. Bad surgeries are done by immoral and sexually immodest women.

In the long run, these interconnected forms of boundary work allow women to take a moral high ground. They adopt a gendered morality that relies on traditional notions of femininity in which women are not supposed to exude hypersexuality or display themselves as overly sexual subjects. Therefore, juxtaposed to pervasive postfeminist rhetoric of female choice and empowerment is an equally pervasive reinforcement of a traditional understanding of femininity—one that tucks away women's sexuality and venerates modesty.

Negotiating "Unnatural" Results

I mutilated myself. I should have just loved myself the way I was.

—ANA MARIE

If I really embraced my uniqueness and I was in love with myself, I feel like I would have been like, "So what? This is me, and this is what makes me beautiful."

—CARLA

Does surgery live up to expectations? If participants desire the natural fake, are they pleased with surgery results? Our findings confirm extant research showing that most cosmetic surgery patients report satisfaction.[1] Even when participants encountered physical complications or expressed disappointment about the look of their postoperative bodies—including dissatisfaction that surgery did not deliver the natural fake—the vast majority framed surgery positively.

In this last data-driven chapter, we examine problems participants encountered and how they responded to them—responses that are in part shaped by status characteristics such as class, race, and ethnicity. We also examine what constitutes successful surgery and illustrate how participants' interpretation of surgery results changes as cultural contexts and bodies change over the life course. Finally, we take a close look at the stories of several participants who struggled with their bodies after surgery, as well as their relationship with cosmetic surgery. Their stories show that, while such wrangling can lead women to challenge hegemonic beauty norms, a negative framing of surgical experiences can also lead to psychological anguish.

Thus, unlike popular media coverage that either showcases surgeries that go dramatically wrong or celebrates over-the-top successful surgical transformation,[2] this chapter brings to light a middle ground. Women's post hoc assessments of cosmetic surgery are not only fluid and shaped by intersecting status characteristics; accompanying narratives of success and empowerment are narratives of discontentment and frustration. Their struggles illustrate that for some women the postoperative body and self require continuous management.

Successful Surgery

Everyday Victories

At the time of their interviews the majority of women we spoke with were content with how surgery turned out.[3] They stated that they did not regret their decision, and many even recommended surgery to others and shared their surgeon's contact information. Jasmine was so ecstatic about her breast augmentation that she intended to celebrate a "boob birthday." Participants were especially pleased with how surgery changed the way they approached everyday activities that had previously caused consternation. For example, Robin described her excitement immediately after having abdominoplasty. Her procedure involved the removal of loose skin and fat in the lower abdominal area: "I'm just excited and happy because I went into the restroom and I wiped. . . . I can wipe without having to lift anything up! [laughs]. I was just very happy."

In particular, clothing became a newfound source of enjoyment. Many participants discussed how clothes shopping and getting dressed were "simpler" after surgery. In their view, they could now comfortably and confidently wear "cute" lacy bras, tank tops, dresses, and shirts. As reported in Chapter 4, before surgery, Taylor cried in changing rooms. After surgery, she, like other participants, no longer dreaded clothes shopping, even saying that it was now enjoyable. Especially for the Californians in our sample, swimsuit season was no longer feared. In short, body consciousness was not a deterrent from participating in everyday activities such as clothes shopping or going to the beach.

Because cosmetic surgery is connected to cultural definitions of womanhood, not unexpectedly many participants mentioned the role of clothing. Postfeminist discourses encourage women to adorn themselves, and the postfeminist woman is supposedly one who is preoccupied with fashion and accessories. Cultural discourses about sexual appeal and power create expectations that women look sexy and powerful, too. We cannot overstate the importance of participants' ability to feel good when clothes shopping and wearing certain clothes. They considered surgery successful for exactly these reasons.

Since cultural discourses construct women as adornments and objects of viewing, particularly for the male gaze,[4] participants connected successful surgery to their appearance in photographs. In the age of social media and ubiquitous smartphones with cameras, successful surgery means no longer shying away from having their picture taken. Lorna, who had jaw surgery at age sixteen, stated emphatically that she was embarrassed to see presurgery photographs. She would tear them up. "I don't like to look at those pictures. There is fugly. There is fucking ugly. And that's how I felt about myself." This is in stark contrast to her postoperative attitude. "I love having attention drawn to my face. I'm constantly taking selfies. Just am! [*laughs*]." Kristen went so far as to delete old pictures off social media accounts. This, she said, would prevent comparisons of her pre- and postoperative body should someone be inclined to make such a comparison. Old photographs serve as a reminder that participants made the right choice by having surgery. Furthermore, the destruction of old photographs serves to aid in stigma management, making it easier for participants to embody the natural fake and pass as surgically unaltered.

In short, armed with their surgically transformed bodies, participants expressed satisfaction with daily victories. With surgery came normalcy, including greater freedom with clothing choices and comfort in front of the camera.

Feeling Good, Motivated, and Proud

Participants also expressed delight that surgery brought psychological changes. As explained in previous chapters, participants have what they believe are laudable psychological motives for surgery.

Dissatisfied with their appearance, they hoped surgery would bring increased confidence and body esteem. Surgery gone right accomplishes this goal by allowing women to feel good, even great, about themselves. Additionally, some participants (such as Lacy) used cosmetic surgery as a turning point that included a changed mind-set. Because surgery is often costly, participants were keen to maintain their postoperative bodies, framing them as an investment in need of protection. Thus, they made renewed commitments to follow physical activity and eating regimens they felt would allow them to maintain or continue to reach their body goals. As an investment in the self, they hoped surgery was not for naught. As Susan put it, she feared "getting big again" and surgery gave her the push she needed to focus on "maintenance."

Caitlin was frank about her goal to implement psychological changes after surgery. After obtaining breast implants, she wanted to "develop [her] personality." She admitted that she "always shied away from people because of social stigma." Surgery, Caitlin believed, provided her with the push she needed to explore parts of her personality she felt were buried because of body insecurity. Like others, she framed successful surgery as a fresh start. Caitlin described her postoperative goals as "trying to make you the best version of you that you can be because you only live once." Similarly, Janet's words capture how a number of participants view cosmetic surgery as a mechanism for change. It is merely one of many tools women use in the project of the self. Janet's narrative was infused with empowerment rhetoric: "[Cosmetic surgery is] empowering because it lets you change what you want to change, become more confident. Then you look better. . . . Have more fun. Be more upbeat."

When surgery went right, participants experienced another less obvious form of psychological value added—pride. Simply, they were proud of themselves for having the courage to go through with surgery. Surgery is not risk-free—physically, financially, or socially. Others talk the talk, but participants walked the walk. So despite her fears and reservations, Elaina went through with rhinoplasty. She recounted an interaction with friends and how it made her feel: "A lot of [my] friends . . . wanted to do stuff like that, but they either didn't have the money, or they were too scared to, [or] they were too embarrassed to make a change. Everyone was like, 'Wow, she had it done?'

I was like, 'Yes.' I felt on top of the world." Even when acknowledging the stigma of cosmetic surgery, participants took pride in taking control of their lives and making the difficult decision to permanently alter their bodies. It takes guts. As Sylvia stated, "There's a lot of people that I know want to do it. I guess they don't have the guts to." Meanwhile, Darla reflected that if she had not had surgery she would "have always wondered, 'What if?'" She took pride in making the decision "without double thinking" herself.

The Body across the Life Course

Although participants affirmed cosmetic surgery's benefits because of these positive life changes, our interviews revealed that the interpretation of surgery results is dynamic across the life course. We spoke with participants between two months and forty-three years after their first surgery, with an average of ten and a half years. Our interviews involved retrospective accounts and, as such, are not technically longitudinal data involving multiple data collection points. Nevertheless, they provide a glimpse into how women think about their bodies over time. So while participants may have expressed satisfaction with surgery immediately following the recovery period, bodies and cultural norms about bodies evolve. Bodies age. They gain and lose weight. What is culturally exalted at one time can be ridiculed at another. These things all influence how women think about their postoperative bodies, potentially leading to the dissipation of satisfaction.

For example, Lena had her first breast surgery in 1995 at age twenty-five. Initially, she was satisfied with her breasts, which she described as double Ds. She joked that what was in at that time was "big hair, big boobs, [and] big earrings." In the mid-1990s, Lena considered her augmented breasts in style. However, as cultural commentators have pointed out, women's body norms are not static.[5] For example, in 1920s America, a boyish, hipless, flat-chested flapper ideal was prominent. By the 1950s, it was replaced by a voluptuous ideal epitomized by Marilyn Monroe. This was followed by the 1960s Twiggy ideal—an embodiment of androgyny and thinness.[6] Lena now believes that the "bigger is better" ideal is no longer "cool." Women's body norms have once again shifted, and this shift affects how she interprets her body: "Here is the other thing that I think a lot about," she said. "If you look back at eighties and nineties fashion magazines or whatever, who did you see? You saw Pamela Anderson, and you saw these skinny [bodies], boobs, big hair, whatever. And look now. Everybody is nice and thin and has just athletic bodies and normal boobs. And I'm like, 'Oh yeah, that would be cool.'" In Lena's opinion, her large breasts are no longer stylish. Dissatisfaction has set in, and she is now contemplating another surgery to make her breasts smaller and more in line with what she considers the current cultural norm.

Physical changes over time can also give rise to disappointment. Lena was not only unhappy that her body now failed to meet current standards of femininity but, like other women who had had breast implants for many years, she was unhappy that her breasts were sagging. She reflected, "I think originally it gave me self-confidence and I was happy about it. Now, I very much regret the size of my chest and them sagging. I was happy as heck, till I was about forty." Hazel's storyline begins the same way. She was initially happy with her augmented breasts. At the time of our interview, she had had them for over ten years. She remarked, however, "Now they've dropped a lot." She planned to deal with the problem within the year: "Well, implants need to be replaced. I'm going to get them replaced and get another breast lift." Even the Food and Drug Administration warns women that breast implants will likely at some point need to be replaced: "Breast implants are not lifetime devices; the longer you have your implants, the more likely it will be for you to have them removed."[7] One study by the Food and Drug Administration indicates that about one in five women have their implants removed (with or without replacement) after ten years.[8]

Weight fluctuations can also affect how participants experience and perceive their postoperative bodies. After three breast surgeries, Charlize was finally pleased with her breasts. But after losing a few pounds, she feels her breasts are disproportionately large for her 5'6", 123-pound body. She commented, "I want them smaller, because I already look at pictures of myself in bikinis, and I'm like, 'Oh, my God, I look like one of those silly skinny people with big boobs.' . . . It used to be cool, but now I just feel very silly. I'm at that point in my life where I'm bummed about it." Like Lena, Charlize believes larger breasts were once fashionable. But now she feels "silly" with what she perceives are disproportionately large and conspicuous breasts. This is a clear violation of the natural fake and possibly an allusion to now looking like the surgical other. These days, she describes herself as "a skeleton with big boobs." She would like to replace her implants but is hesitant to go back under the knife. She is deterred by Joan Rivers's death. The comedienne and actress died of cerebral hypoxia (lack of oxygen to the brain) during a minor throat procedure. Charlize joked with a tinge of reservation, "I'm like, I might be stuck with big boobs until I'm like a hundred! I have no idea."

In contrast to Charlize, whose weight loss led to discontentment, dissatisfaction set in for Penelope after weight gain. She too was thrilled at first with her breast augmentation, saying that she's "always been a little hippy" and that surgery "balanced" her and made her more proportionate. But these days she admits to being heavier than she was at age twenty-six, when she had surgery: "I'm turning sixty-two in three months. After menopause and all that, I'm probably packing like an extra twenty-five or thirty pounds. . . . So now my boobs look bigger and I hate it! [laughs heartily]. . . . Because the bigger you are, the bigger they are. It's like, 'Eew.'" She continued to complain that her "boobs have really dropped [laughs]." But unlike Charlize's, Penelope's disappointment was not intense enough to prompt further surgery. Although stating she "hate[s]" her large breasts, she said, "This is probably it. . . . I probably need a lift, but I'm not going to do it. No, I'm happy with what I've got going on." Notably, Penelope's choice of the word "need" illustrates the power of the beauty mandate and the way participants often see cosmetic surgery as necessary.

Bodies and cultural norms are dynamic, which make experiences of the body dynamic. With time, some participants tended toward dissatisfaction. Changing beauty ideals led them to redefine their postsurgical bodies as undesirable. Weight loss or gain resulted in breasts appearing disproportionately obvious and large, an aesthetic letdown that is antithetical to a quintessential attribute of the natural fake—inconspicuousness. Thus, despite the boundary work that criticized these types of outcomes, some participants admitted that their postoperative bodies soon became unruly. The fluidity of both cultural norms and the physical body means there is always the possibility of seeing characteristics of the surgical other in oneself.

Surgery Complications and Letdowns

Overall, participants framed cosmetic surgery positively. Yet this does not mean they were satisfied with *all* aspects of surgery. They shared numerous stories about their struggles with recovery, including unanticipated side effects. Their stories show that surgery is sometimes disappointing and does not always live up to its billing. They experienced physical complications and aesthetic letdowns. These two themes are not mutually exclusive; physical problems after surgery can certainly have aesthetic consequences.

Physical Complications and Side Effects

Infections and Nerve Damage

Cosmetic surgery is invasive surgery insofar as it involves skin breakage and therefore carries health risks. Areas around surgery sites can become infected, and body parts can become tingly or numb from nerve damage.[9] Participants reported all these problems. For example, after having a trunk lift, Barbara was rehospitalized with a MRSA infection.[10] She described intense rounds of antibiotic treatment delivered intravenously. The infection lengthened the healing process considerably. She admitted she was terrified: "It did take more time out from what I originally planned, and the rehospitalization scared the hell out of me!"

Lena detected an infection about a month after her second breast surgery. She was vacationing in Hawaii when she sensed something was wrong. "All of a sudden I have stuff leaking through the sutures," she recalled. She immediately called her doctor, asking, "Am I going to die?" Because she was not flying home for another two weeks, the doctor called in a prescription and told her not to get into the salt water. During the rest of her vacation, she was continuously releasing a lot of "body fluid." "It was disgusting," she said with a cringe. Upon returning home, she visited her doctor, who determined the implant was in fact infected. However, because he wanted the area to heal before putting in another implant, for three months Lena had what she described as a "deflated balloon" on one side of her chest. During this healing period she was "self-conscious," stating candidly, "It was awful."

Unlike Barbara's and Lena's one-time infections, Elaina's postoperative infection was recurring. For about a decade after having ear surgery the skin behind her ear became irritated. "Maybe seven to ten years, something around there, I would get an infection. . . . It was like a boil and it would bleed." She recalled going to a dermatologist who told her it was a "pimple or something." However given the tenacity of the irritation, she soon became skeptical of this diagnosis. The area "would always get infected." Eventually, Elaina consulted another doctor who, upon probing the area with a "little tweezer, took out a piece of string that was left there." Since removing this string, which she deduced the surgeon left in the incision site, Elaina has not experienced further problems in the area. However, she began "having nightmares where I would dream that my ears would fall off." Even though the nightmares have gone away, the experience, she said, left her "traumatized."

Other participants reported a loss of physical sensation. Despite being informed by her surgeon about this possible side effect, Lavanna's inability to feel certain sensations in her abdominal area unnerved her: "The doctor said the feeling really doesn't come back, anywhere from five to seven years. Sometimes he said it just won't. I think that's the scariest part. I can feel a fly land on me, but if it did something—bit me—I probably wouldn't feel that. I can just tingle, but I can't feel nothing harsh." Lorna too, after jaw surgery, lost sensation in her face. She was made aware of this during one incident in a public setting: "I'm completely numb right here [points at her jaw area]. So ranch dressing will fall down my face and I have no idea. And my husband, when we first were dating, he would laugh and would let me sit there in the restaurant." Since this incident, Lorna has made her spouse alert her if she has something on her face that should not be there: "So now he promises. But I have no feeling here."

A few participants had a hard time describing the postoperative sensations they felt. After having breast augmentation, a body lift, and liposuction, Jasmine now experiences numbness, as well as what she described as an "odd feeling." She put it this way: "What's funny is, . . . once that stopped being stinging from where the incision was, it gets numb because they cut through all your nerves. . . . Some portions I can feel, and some I can't. And it's all surface numbness, so I still get sensations like getting itches or feeling heat and warmth, but I can't feel something actually touching my skin. It's very weird. And it's only on certain parts of my body." Similarly, Martha discussed how after her face-lift, abdominoplasty, and liposuction, she had itching and tingling in areas where she did not have surgery. She invented her own term to capture these feelings, which reflects how they come and go: "I still have itching and tingling. It's like it flipped a switch in my body—an itch switch. . . . I itched in places I didn't have lipo. It was really peculiar. Yeah, and it went everywhere." While "it's not nearly as bad as it once was," these days her body continues to unpredictably activate this "itch switch."

Breast Implants That Harden, Rupture, Wrinkle, and Slosh

Participants who had breast implants cited a number of unique problems. The Food and Drug Administration identifies specific risks related to breast implants such as hardening, deflation, rupture, and wrinkling.[11] Participants reported all these. For example, the breast area or implant can harden over time, a side effect known as capsular contracture.[12] This was Jessica's experience. She was happy with her decision to have cosmetic surgery for quite some time—"about ten, fifteen, twenty years." Then her implants turned into "rocks in a sock." She elaborated, "They became rock hard, like, almost golf balls." For this reason, several decades after her first surgery, she went back under the knife to replace the hardened implants.

Other participants, such as Heather, experienced implant rupture. After ten years, her saline implant ruptured. She was left, she said, feeling "abnormal" once again. "So I'm walking around feeling disfigured. I mean I felt freakish before any surgeries and, . . . now here I am walking around and I have something broken in my body." Because the leakage was not life threatening and her surgeon was not immediately available, she waited over a month in this "abnormal" state. Notably, even participants who did not experience ruptures expressed anxiety about this possible side effect. Sarah said, "I had chosen to get silicone implants, so then I had this fear, 'Oh my gosh, it's leaking. I'm sick.'" Rebecca disclosed a similar concern, "I'm always afraid that it's leaking."

Charlize's saline implants leaked after three years. With the leakage was also another problem with the implant area—wrinkling. She described it this way: "My skin is so thin, and because I was a 32AA, . . . you could literally see ripples on the top of my chest . . . because it's like a water bag. . . . And so the saline bag kind of left indentions, so I couldn't even wear bathing suits or anything. It looked horrible." To fix the leakage and wrinkling, her surgeon replaced the saline implant with teardrop silicone implants, which Charlize also did not like because they "hung kinda long and skinny." "They looked so funny," she said with a chuckle. Still, she kept these teardrop silicone implants for about seven years. Then she went through a divorce and received some money. Not wanting to be single with breasts she disliked, she found a new surgeon who put in round silicone implants. As mentioned previously, she was initially content with these implants. However, after losing weight she started struggling again with the look of her breasts, believing they look disproportionately large for her body.

Finally, Sarah and Leanne experienced sloshing implants. Whereas Sarah consulted her surgeon and elected not to redo her breast implants, the sloshing bothered Leanne so much that she went back under the knife to replace them. For Leanne, the sloshing also came with the same sort of puckering Charlize described. Leanne explained, "I didn't go back for bigger and better. I went back because I could hear them sloshing. I didn't like the feel. If you bend over to tie your shoe or whatever, the gravity pull on your body, it kinda looked like the side of a pool raft. You know, how it puckers, and you could see that. . . . And I just, I kept thinking I could hear them. Oh, that's just weird."

Aesthetic Letdowns

Physical complications sometimes require medical attention and follow-up surgery. Aesthetic disappointments bring about a different set of concerns. Participants discussed how they did not like the appearance of scars and how surgery did not live up to their aesthetic expectations.

Scars

Scars are blemishes that violate feminine aesthetic norms and run counter to the natural fake. Cosmetic surgery scars, identified as such, signify to others that one has purposely surgically altered the body in the pursuit of beauty. Even the best cosmetic surgeons will leave traces of their work.[13] The American Board of Cosmetic Surgery recognizes this, writing that "scarring is a necessary aspect of many surgeries." The board encourages patients to protect incisions from the sun, keep the area clean, and use ointments recommended by doctors to minimize the appearance of scars.[14] While surgery may seem to be a one-and-done deal, it requires ongoing personal upkeep to maintain or optimize results.

The extent that participants thought their surgical scars were noticeable, and thus needed accounting for and management, varied. Some participants emphasized that their scars were barely visible. For example, Hanna said, "They're in the crease of my armpit and you can't even see them." Lacy described her scar as the "size of my thumbnail," commenting that "it kinda looks like a stretch mark." A few participants acknowledged that their light skin tone helped. Casey, who identifies as white, said, "The scars were really not too much of an issue because I'm so pale. . . . That's one of the many reasons why I stay out of the sun." She is aware that a suntan might diminish this advantage and, thus, consciously avoids sun exposure. Similarly, Jasmine, who also identifies as white, agreed with her doctor that her skin tone makes her scars less noticeable. "He [her doctor] said if I had darker skin, the scars probably would have been more prominent." She continued, "They're not that bad. And they fade."

In this way, scars have a racial or ethnic element to them. They can be more noticeable on people with darker skin tones. However, this is not to say that participants with darker skin tones were overly concerned with scars or that sun avoidance was a concern only for white participants. For example, Taylor, who identifies as Hispanic, also avoided the sun, fearing her scars would become more visible. She admitted to "freaking out," thinking, "I'm going to have this scar forever!" But about a year after surgery, it started to fade. She was pleased to recount a recent experience: "I was shopping for a bathing suit, and I was like, 'Oh, the scars I was worried about, they're not even there anymore!'" Similarly, Kristen, who identifies as black, said she was "impressed with the scar" and how it faded. Even though she explicitly said she didn't like her scar and actively managed it, she also insisted "it is fading" and said, "I know eventually it will be gone."

In contrast, some participants voiced that their scars bothered them quite a bit. Susan stated with a tinge of sarcasm, "The scarring is huge. . . . I don't plan on doing beauty queen pageants where I have to wear a bikini or anything like that. But it's just the fact that it was from hip to hip. I think that just kinda freaked me out." Similarly, Kali's concerns about her abdominoplasty scar illustrate how scars must be accounted for. After surgery, she found herself subconsciously rubbing the scar. She described the area as "really itchy," and nearly six months after surgery she is still "super aware" of it. To compound matters, one day she showed her coworkers her scar. She described their reaction: "And the guys were like, 'Wow, how are you going to have sex?'" At first she thought, "What do you mean, what am I going to do?" She continued, "That's when it dawned on me that guys might care," particularly those her age, in their mid-twenties. Unlike the scars she has from playing sports, this scar is different. Kali reflected, "I have so many scars from sports that a scar is a scar, but it's [this abdominal scar] a very intimate[ly] located scar. . . . It's not like a cleat ripped up my knee, and you can see it, and I have a good story about it." To her dismay her scar now prompts the need to account for cosmetic surgery. She feels she must justify this elective work to potential sexual partners.

Surgery That Fails to Meet Aesthetic Expectations
Along with scarring, some participants were disappointed with how their bodies looked after surgery. They had initially turned to surgery to transform body parts they deemed unsightly, and sometimes surgery failed to achieve this objective. Disappointment can be immediate or set in over time. As illustrated earlier in this chapter, new beauty norms mean a reinterpretation of what is desirable. Gravity inevitably takes its toll. Weight loss or gain and aging occur. Aesthetic letdowns can also accompany physical complications, as was the case with Heather's and Lena's deflated breasts.

The aesthetic letdowns participants experienced came in many forms. After surgery, Elaina felt her ears were still uneven. She said,

"See, I think one is still a little bit more out than the other one. I don't know if you can tell, one is fatter than the other." Susan too felt that the procedures on her abdomen left her uneven, specifically that the right side stuck out more than the left. In her eyes, it was not something one could miss: "It sticks out. It's obvious that it's uneven." Meanwhile, Darla, whom we spoke to about three months after she had rhinoplasty, felt that her nose was still deviated. She described it as a "waiting game." Her doctor informed her that her full transformation would be a yearlong process as her face continued to heal. In the meantime, she manipulated her nose daily in hopes of seeing more pleasing results. Vanessa too was disappointed that one breast was "a little bit lower." Although conceding it was minor, she said, "It bothers me to the point where I'm going to get them redone."

Alongside lack of symmetry, some participants framed aesthetic disappointments in terms of surgeons doing too little. They wanted more dramatic change. Nadine, who said she would not have liposuction again, was lukewarm about how she looked after surgery: "Visually, to me, I looked the same. I was like, I still have a belly. It was weird. Even though I knew it wasn't going to be hard rock or anything. I don't know. It was okay." Hanna was more vocal. She was "very happy" with her breast augmentation but not her rhinoplasty. Regarding the latter, "Yeah, I wasn't happy at all. . . . It wasn't as extreme as I wanted." Similarly, Kali was upset that her mini abdominoplasty created a flat lower abdominal area but left a bulge above her belly button. These results were frustrating for her given what she felt she sacrificed. She said, "The pain and the emotional part was so extreme that I wish the benefit was more to what I think the cost was." Other participants also interpreted surgery results through a cost-benefit lens. For example, Hazel's experiences were similar to Hanna's. She was thrilled with her breast augmentation—even saying, "They looked amazing. They were perfect ten breasts"—but was dissatisfied with rhinoplasty. She was angry because she worked hard to save up for the procedure. For the money, she wanted greater returns. Her reaction upon seeing her nose for the first time after surgery was "I wanted my nose to be more pronounced, more distinct here. He took off the bandages. I've never been so upset in my life. My nose looked the exact same. I had to spend my babysitting money and work money to pay for it! It wasn't covered under insurance."

Unexpected Lifestyle Changes

Alongside physical complications and aesthetic letdowns, a handful of participants—mostly women who had breast surgery—reported that surgery resulted in unanticipated lifestyle changes. First, they reported experiencing physical pain and discomfort, even long after the recovery period. For instance, after three breast augmentations, Charlize said she now experiences chronic pain in her shoulders and back. Because breast surgery stretched the skin on Ana Marie's chest, the area continues to hurt years later. Carla reported that she did not have back pain immediately after surgery but developed it about two years after. She attributes this pain to her breast surgery. After abdominoplasty, Lavanna described her stomach area as persistently "uncomfortable."

Second, while none of the participants described this pain and discomfort as unmanageable or life threatening, it was still burdensome and impinged on their lifestyles, including their ability to exercise. For example, Hanna and Kerrie are no longer able to do pull-ups or push-ups during their workouts. For Hanna, it was because of the pain she felt ("I can't do push-ups. For some reason, it hurts, it separates them"), while for Kerrie it was because of an odd sensation ("I can't use as much chest muscle. . . . It's not painful. I just feel my chest splitting, so whenever I feel that I stop"). Kali, Ana Marie, and Sarah reported that they were no longer able to run. Kali felt her stomach was too stiff. Before surgery, she used to wake up and run a couple of miles but is now unable to because "there's still a weird tugging." Ana Marie now turns to biking or swimming because, she said, "When I run, I feel like they [her breast implants] are uncomfortably pushing back against my ribs." For Sarah, it was a matter of not being able to find the support she needed to run. She eventually gave up: "I can't run anymore because I can't find a right sports bra that makes me comfortable enough to run."

So while participants expressed newfound joy over their ability to wear feminine clothing, they struggled to find undergarments that provided sufficient breast support. Hanna was able to do her workout routine (sans pushups) only if she wears two sports bras. After surgery, participants emphasized the need for greater breast support even outside the gym. Ana Marie finds her implants "so heavy" that she must wear a push-up bra every day, which she says provides more support.

Finally, two participants reported having recurring sleep problems, which they attribute to their surgeries. Since her surgery, Carla wakes up in pain from sleeping on her stomach, even though she has slept this way since she was a baby. After surgery, Charlize finds it uncomfortable to sleep on her side and adjusts by using an additional pillow for breast support. While these lifestyle changes may seem minor, both exercise and sleep are essential for a woman's healthy lifestyle.

Responding to Complications and Letdowns

Participants responded to these setbacks by turning to management strategies. *Physical* management strategies involve bodily change or manipulation. Participants used these strategies to deal with physical complications that needed medical attention, but they also used them to deal with aesthetic disappointments. With physical management, participants turned to medical experts to correct perceived problems or used props or the body itself to conceal or redirect attention away from aesthetic disappointments. In contrast, participants used *psychological* management strategies mainly to cope with aesthetic disappointments. These strategies involve a cognitive reframing that allows participants to interpret their decision to have surgery as empowering rather than as something they might regret.

Physical Management

Fix It

An obvious solution to a perceived problem related to cosmetic surgery is to have a surgeon fix it. This is sensible because cosmetic surgeons are trained and skilled experts. Moreover, certain physical complications require immediate medical attention. Of our forty-six participants, nine had a second procedure of the same nature to address the side effects or results of a previous surgery. So when participants such as Heather, Leanne, Charlize, and Jessica experienced rupturing, sloshing, puckering, or hardening of their implants, they all sought medical attention. After bringing their concerns to their surgeon's attention, they replaced problematic implants. Problem solved. Charlize, who had three breast surgeries, used this strategy to fix a leak as well as an implant she did not think was attractive. Similarly, Hazel, who redid her nose several times and was experiencing sagging implants at the time of her interview, stated without hesitation that she planned to have her breasts redone.

Certainly, this strategy is classed. Time and money are needed for repairs. Follow-up surgeries are not without costs. When Leanne replaced her sloshing and puckering implants, the doctor agreed not to charge her "doctor's fees." But she still had to pay "for the replacement implants and hospital time"—costs she placed at about $4,000. For Jessica, replacing hardened implants in 2014 cost her about $7,000—$4,000 more than she paid for her original implants in 1972. Charlize's first breast surgery was about $3,500; the second about $4,500; and the third about $5,000. Because income corresponds to race and ethnicity in both the U.S. population and our sample,[15] this physical management strategy was adopted mostly by our white participants from middle- and upper-socioeconomic backgrounds.

This prevalent fix-it mentality is consistent with participants' mind-set that cosmetic surgery is a relatively safe and well-established scientific tool that women should take advantage of. In their view, cosmetic surgery exists to help women achieve their desired selves. They see it as a solution to the problem of body dissatisfaction. Even when it becomes the cause of further body consternation, they enthusiastically return to it. Unlike Charlize who, after three surgeries, voiced reservations about future surgery because of Joan Rivers's untimely death, the major deterrent to this fix-it strategy is not the fear of potential health risks or dying under the knife. Rather, it is the cost. Thus, Vanessa, Ana Marie, and Carla—all women of color who were disappointed with their postoperative breasts—held off on "corrective" surgery because of their financial situations. In the same breath that she uttered dismay with surgery, Vanessa said, "If I had the money, I probably would redo it."

Conceal It

Obvious scars are blatant violations of the natural fake, and participants made conscious efforts to conceal them. This strategy was particularly evident with abdominoplasty patients whose scars were hip to hip. To conceal these scars, participants reported using makeup, "scar serum," and fade creams. They mentioned pharmaceutical products such as Mederma, a topical cream that is applied daily to reduce the appearance of scars, along with makeup products such as Dermablend—a line of makeup products manufactured by L'Oréal. Dermablend products, as the manufacturer professes, are "recommended by dermatologists and plastic surgeons worldwide" and provide "natural-looking coverage for minor to major skin imperfections."[16]

Kristen's primary strategy for dealing with scars was concealment. She had breast augmentation, abdominoplasty, and liposuction. She was not concerned about the scar underneath her breasts. She thought it was discreet and had faded. "But I have a scar that goes across my tummy really low. It's still visible," she said. Her preoperative research made her aware that she would be left with a remarkable scar. She weighed her options and concluded a scar was an acceptable trade-off for a flatter stomach. Besides, she believed clothing could be used to conceal the scar: "I knew with a tummy tuck you would have a scar, but I was like, 'Stuff I wear, you won't see it,' and I want to have a flat tummy, so I just went forward with it."

After surgery, she admitted that she would now "sit a certain way, or I'll position myself where it's not visible." She will also not wear clothing, such as string bikinis, that draws attention to her scar. About a year and a half after her surgery, she was still looking into a "surgical remover" (i.e., laser treatment) and using fade creams and makeup. She was pleased with Dermablend and said, "It's meant to cover up tattoos but it covers up my scars. . . . It covers up so you can't tell. That's nice." However, she conceded that makeup as a scar management strategy has it limits. Our conversation continued:

> KRISTEN: Some people take showers with guys. I don't do that. I'm not there yet because that scar would be there. You could put the little Dermablend cover-up stuff, but it's going to wash off. I don't even want the question. I don't want them to know I had plastic surgery.
>
> INTERVIEWER: That's right, you said you don't disclose your surgery.

KRISTEN: Yeah, and if they see my tummy scar, they're going to suspect my boobs too.

For Kristen, concealing the scar on her stomach requires ongoing management. To hide it, she positions her body, avoids certain clothing, and uses fade cream and makeup. She fears others, especially men she is in a relationship with, might discover she had cosmetic surgery in her stomach area. This is exacerbated by a fear they might then deduce she had breast augmentation surgery. Yet counterintuitively, Kristen's ongoing efforts, which involve emotional and physical energy, do not correlate with a negative attitude toward cosmetic surgery. When asked about her all-around sentiment about her surgeries, she replied enthusiastically that they are "completely successful. One hundred percent!" Despite requiring daily management to conceal her scars, they do not take away from her overall enjoyment of her postoperative body.

It was not uncommon for participants to use clothing to conceal scars. It is an easy and accessible strategy. For example, when Heather's implant ruptured, she immediately resorted to wearing loose T-shirts. Participants not only avoid clothing that might reveal surgical scars but also ensure that clothing is positioned to cover them. Lavanna said, "When I'm in my house I don't care. And then when I'm outside, I'm usually wearing clothes that you can't see it [the scar]. It's when I'm wearing clothes that you can see [the scar] that I get a little self-conscious." She continued to describe how she is quite mindful of her scar, particularly at the swimming pool:

LAVANNA: Over the years it's gotten lighter and lighter. So I've noticed that. At first it was dark and it scared me. My sister kept wanting me to wear my stomach out, and I didn't feel comfortable. And I was like, no. Because I was worried about what if my clothes, like, mess up and somebody sees my scar. Before surgery, I never thought I'd be worrying about some scar. Now, after surgery, I am worried about some scar. I'm worried about how my clothes fall.

INTERVIEWER: Does this prevent you from wearing a bikini?

LAVANNA: I make sure my bikini covers it. And when I'm playing, I still even check to make sure when I get out of the water.

Lavanna is mindful of her scar, and when she cannot conceal it, she feels self-conscious. Like Kristen's, Lavanna's management is ongoing. And like Kristen, even though it is a daily burden, Lavanna said this scar and its accompanying management are not overly bothersome. It does not change her overall evaluation of cosmetic surgery. In her words, her surgeries are a resounding "success." She is now considering breast augmentation and will factor in how the scar will look before making a decision: "I'll go online and look at different scarring. I will have the appearance of bigger breasts, but I will look at my scars as constant. . . . Which one do I really want? Do I want the appearance that I have bigger breasts and know that there's going to be scars? Or do I just leave it alone and be comfortable with what I have?" By the end of our conversation, she had voiced certainty that she will eventually have breast augmentation.

Redirect Attention from It

A handful of participants used another physical management strategy to deal with scars. They diverted attention away from them. For example, Robin was considering a tattoo if her abdominoplasty scar did not fade further. She felt it would redirect attention from it: "I might try tattoos. That's one thing I've thought about, maybe along my scar or above. . . . I might consider having some kind of decoration, kinda like just basically an eye-catcher to distract from that [the scar] that would be cute in a bathing suit." Barbara adopted a similar strategy, but her goal was to deflect focus from the entire surgery site. After her operation, she consciously made a few fashion changes so her surgery would be less conspicuous. She said, "I had more redirection. I got my hair cut. I got new glasses." These new props were effective at drawing attention to her face rather than her stomach area.

Yet similar to concealment, redirection has its limits. When discussing the impact of surgery on intimate relations, Barbara admitted, "There was still a lot of shame about it. Rather than a pannus [excess skin and tissue at the lower abdomen][17] to explain, now there was a scar to explain. Either way, you had to go through the rocky portion of the story to get to the reality of the truth, and you had to figure out how much you trust them, how much they're going to be in your life long term, and how much you actually reveal." For Barbara, she had merely traded one stigma (excess skin and tissue) for

another (an abdominal scar signifying surgery). Ultimately, concealment and redirection still require accounting for surgery, which in
her case meant carefully choosing whom she could trust.

Psychological Management

Alongside physical management strategies, participants used several
psychological management strategies to downplay aesthetic letdowns.
These strategies involve a positive reframing of surgery that minimizes cognitive dissonance—the experience of conflicting values and
beliefs that lead to psychological discomfort.[18] Sure, their postoperative body was not exactly what they had envisioned, but they reasoned
that, all in all, it was not too bad. It is plausible that their positive attitude was because their physical management strategies and cognitive reframing helped neutralize disappointment. It is also plausible
that they had an optimistic mentality from the outset that led them
to seek out and use such strategies.[19]

First, participants reframed an aesthetic disappointment accompanying surgery as the lesser of two evils. We saw how Lavanna opted
for a flatter stomach knowing there would be a scar, and Barbara
preferred the stigma of a cosmetic surgery scar over the stigma of
excess skin. Second, participants adopted a to-be-expected attitude.
As reported in Chapter 4, in contrast to the imaginary surgical other
who is unrealistic, participants did not expect perfection. For example, Penelope was fine with the scar on top of her left eyelid, saying,
"It comes with the territory." Even though Elaina felt her ears were
still somewhat uneven after surgery, she said she did not regret having the procedure. These days she even pulls her hair back to reveal
her altered ears, stressing everyone has flaws: "Now I can pick up
my hair and not worry about it. Even if I stick it back, I'm like, 'Hey,
everybody has a little flaw here and there.' Now, I've come to accept
that." Lily too, who was not entirely pleased with her postoperative
nose, still accepts the results. She said, "I feel like I could have gotten
a straighter nose, and even a little bit thinner, and had more tissue
taken out at the end of my nose. But I don't think I would go back to
have it, not enough to where I would want a revision." In this way,
participants rationalize aesthetic letdowns, including underwhelm-
ing results, as something they can live with. Consequently, the results

do not cause tremendous psychological grief. Relatedly, participants downplayed aesthetic problems, simply saying they were not that bad. They were convinced that scars would fade with time, laser treatments, and ointments. They believed, as did Darla, who was waiting to see progress after having rhinoplasty, that aesthetically pleasing results would eventually materialize as their bodies continued to heal.

When Surgery Goes Wrong: Surgery as Oppressive

Despite tales of physical complications and aesthetic disappointment, only four of our forty-six participants expressed serious concern about their decision to have surgery or framed their surgeries negatively. Chapter 4 covers Rebecca's story. This chapter closes by turning to the stories of Ana Marie, Lena, and Carla. Their narratives underscore how class and social networks shape responses to cosmetic surgery and outlooks on beauty. They also call attention to the psychological anguish that can accompany cosmetic surgery when surgery does not produce envisioned outcomes.

Self-Mutilation and Self-Loathing

We met Ana Marie when she was twenty-seven. At the time, she was working on her college degree and as a part-time waitress. She had been married for five years and had a young daughter. At age nine, she had moved from Colombia to the United States. Ana Marie had thought about having breast surgery since age fifteen and went through with it at age twenty-five. She said her preoperative body looked like a "snake" and a "little girl." While she was content with her face, she wanted "everything to look nice." She wanted "the whole package." She yearned to feel more feminine and sexy, a desire she said was driven in part by her ethnic background. "I hated the way I looked. I thought I looked like a surfboard, especially in my culture." She explained, "In Hispanic culture, they like curviness, and I think I let it get to me too much. I got too conscious about it." She felt people made fun of her small breasts—"my culture is like that; even my grandmother, she's criticized other people that don't have breasts." She also believed Hispanic men have only one ideal of femininity. "They like big boobs," she stated. This ideal, she said, is "even in the mind-set of the girls." Like her Colombian cousins, she wanted "big boobs, too. Not super big, but just to look nice."

Her choice of surgeon was driven largely by funds. Despite thinking about surgery for ten years, she did minimal research. She turned to the internet and typed "breast augmentation" into a search engine. She then visited the websites of three surgeons the search engine returned. Because consultations were about $100, she said she could not afford multiple in-person consultations. Consequently, she chose the surgeon "that was marketed the best online." When asked to elaborate, she explained that he had a "Black Diamond" certification and was supposedly ranked in the top 2 percent of surgeons in the state. However, in hindsight, she reflected, "It doesn't mean that he's the best." Her lack of funds, together with her enthusiasm about having breast surgery, seems to have clouded her judgment. She said, "I was so excited about getting it done that I didn't really stop and think about it." (She also admitted that she was less concerned about the general standard of care she would receive in the United States compared with Colombia, saying that there is greater industry regulation here.) As an incentive, the surgeon she selected offered her a $1,000 discount if she had surgery in the summer (shortly after her consultation). In the end, surgery cost Ana Marie $5,650. She paid a $500 deposit and is now making monthly payments. In retrospect, she believes this is "not a wise thing to do. When you get it done, you should have all the money in your pocket [and] pay upfront."

Before surgery, Ana Marie had little contact with her surgeon. During her first consultation, she said her surgeon informed her that implants are safe, and she described her ideal breasts to him. She recounted, "When I went to the first consultation, I told him that I wanted it to look natural, because I've seen some girls looked like they have soccer balls on their chest." He then recommended that the incision be made around the areola. However, she said, "I was scared because I was, like, 'This is a very sensitive part.' Then it would probably hurt. The recovery would probably be a lot." So she asked for "under the breast." Ana Marie felt he "didn't give me much time" during this initial consultation, and she was just "left with his assistant to try on sizes." She complained, "She wasn't even a nurse." To her surprise, during the second appointment, her surgeon was not even in the office. She speculated that he was at another one of his three office locations. Once again, she spent time with his assistant trying on different implant sizes.

On the day of surgery, she learned more about the incision and how scars might be more visible with an incision under the breast. She broached the subject with her surgeon. "He didn't let me finish," she recalled. From her perspective, he interrupted and told her, "No, you already decided that you wanted under the breast, and it's going to be under the breast." She considered calling off the surgery but was deterred by the cost. She clarified, "If you cancel it, they charge you $500 just for canceling it." She believes her physical condition played a role in not putting up a fight: "I was also too weak because you cannot eat before the surgery, and it was already one o'clock and I was really weak. I just went along with him."

Surgery failed to achieve Ana Marie's objectives. She wanted to feel feminine and essentially requested the natural fake from her surgeon. But surgery resulted in disproportionately large breasts she now describes as "heavy," "sagging," and "drooping." She complained that they "don't meet and they're too low." She is upset that she is not able to get cleavage when she wears a tank top. Her curviness, she lamented, is revealed only when she is completely naked. In her mind, they are also "too pointy, almost like cones," "too protruded," and look "like volcanoes." Her surgeon informed her that "he couldn't make them meet," but she said, "I've seen other girls that are like my size, and they have better boob jobs." Her aunt had had breast augmentation in Colombia two decades ago, and Ana Marie thought she would look better than her because "medicine has come a long way since twenty years." Yet with resignation, she quipped, "No, unfortunately no." Her dislike of her implants is compounded by her belief that they make her look older.

Ana Marie is self-conscious about her postoperative breasts. She thinks people she meets speculate about her breasts: "Are they wondering if they're fake or real?" Her spouse, who Ana Marie said is just trying to be honest with her, told her, "I think they're just too big for your body. . . . I think they [people in general] look at you because it's not usual that you see big boobs on a small person." She continued, "I wish they were smaller. . . . I was self-conscious before the surgery and now I'm self-conscious again." A year and a half after surgery, she is still reminded daily of her surgery. The silicone feels heavy: "The skin, it's like it's not sturdy enough to really support the implant. . . . It's like it's tired of holding it." Her entire body had to get used to the weight: "I had problems with my spine getting used to it, because your whole body has to get used to it. Your legs have to get used to carrying the extra weight because it's silicone . . . gel [and] . . . heavy." When standing up, she finds herself pushing back her shoulders to adjust to the weight. To prevent further discomfort, she is also careful not to bump into things. This is quite a challenge because she waits tables. The implants also affect her intimate life. She has to "tell him [her spouse] to be careful because if there's too much pressure they start hurting." They affect her exercise patterns, too. She used to enjoy running but is not able to now because the implants push up against her ribs. She resorts these days to biking and swimming.

In short, surgery was a big letdown for Ana Marie. She wanted the natural fake. She wanted to look feminine and sexy. She wanted to feel good about herself. Instead, cosmetic surgery has left her "depressed" and with the same feelings of self-consciousness she had before going under the knife.

Ana Marie struggles with her decision to have surgery. Without reservation, she says she regrets it. "Why did I do this to myself? It's almost like I mutilated myself. I should have just loved myself the way I was, and I felt like I betrayed myself because I did this. If I had loved myself more, I wouldn't have harmed my body this way." While she says her grandmother supported her during the surgery, "she never told me to love myself the way I was." She said that she wished she had had someone to talk to who would have helped with her self-esteem. Physical appearance, she admitted, was always important to her, but her cosmetic surgery experience has her rethinking this priority. To compound matters, she regrets having to make monthly payments— ongoing reminders of her decision. "I should have used my money for something better, more meaningful than this, more worthwhile, like a vacation or having fun with my family." She continues, "Now, I'm wiser with money." Her experiences have allowed her to "mature" and "put her feet on the ground."

Ana Marie is considering a second surgery to address her dissatisfaction. But she does not have the money. "I'm broke right now," she said. Because she is concerned that her large breasts are conspicuous and signify to others that they are surgically altered, she minimizes her use of makeup. In her view, she was aiming for "natural-looking breasts" but now has these "fake things." "I try to be natural because, since I have these fake things, I don't want to look too fake with too much makeup."

Ana Marie holds an unfavorable view of her surgeon: "I don't know if it's all of the doctors' places that they do that, but I regret going there." She continued, "I should have just waited another year when I had more money so I could see different doctors before I decided." In addition, she suspects he might have been tired when he operated on her "because he had operated on someone else before me . . . from nine until noon. Then, they have to clean the operating room, and then it was me." In retrospect, she felt his experience was inadequate, explaining, "Now that I think about it, I don't think eleven years is enough experience." She was also upset that she was in the dark about how tough the recovery process would be. The doctor gave her little information, she said. His staff even said to her, "Oh, this is a fun surgery."

She is critical of her surgeon, but Ana Marie also blames herself. She rebukes herself for making a request that she felt might have led to confusion: "I didn't explain myself very well to him. I didn't even bring a picture. So it's my fault that I didn't end up looking like I wanted." She says she will "never forget that I have these things." Her struggle to achieve self-love and forgiveness is ongoing. She wants others to know about her experiences so that they do not make the same mistakes she did.

Unable to Escape an Oppressive Beauty Culture

We met Lena when she was forty-four. She was a stay-at-home mom raising two teenage boys. At the time of her interview, she had been divorced for about five years. She had her first cosmetic surgery at eighteen. The rhinoplasty was a high school graduation gift from her parents. As a teenager, she felt her schoolmates had cuter and smaller noses. So she did what she thought all teenage girls who lived in Orange County did when they were disappointed with a body part—she asked her parents for cosmetic surgery. Her nose did not cause her much grief, she admits. Instead, getting cosmetic surgery was "in vogue." She conceded, "It was subtle and unnecessary, but everybody was doing it." In this area of Southern California, it was "boob jobs for sixteenth birthdays and nose jobs."[20]

Her nose job was followed by breast augmentation at age twenty-five. She had recently married and had yet to give birth to her boys. She was living in an affluent coastal city near the Pacific Ocean and wanted a certain look: "We were going to clubs and doing this and doing that. It was purely, like, it was how I wanted to look." Her mom had firm recommendations for Lena's breast augmentation. She had done two rhinoplasties, a face-lift, and breast surgery (to increase her bra size to about a full B). She advised Lena to increase her breast size to a maximum of C. However, Lena rejected this advice, saying that what was in at that time was "big boobs." She opted for saline implants that were the equivalent of double Ds. Her surgeon was supportive, and she even recalled him saying, "Let's go big or go home." "Total cosmetic surgeon, you know," she joked.

About a decade later and after nursing two children, Lena was not satisfied with the look of her breasts. She also felt that her breast "texture was different." So she consulted a surgeon to have them lifted, as well as reduced. However, during the consultation he informed her that her skin had stretched, which would mean "big scars." Consequently, when she went under the knife for a third time at age thirty-six, she kept the same size implant (although she replaced the original saline implant with a silicone one). It was this second implant that became infected when she vacationed in Hawaii.

Despite this infection, Lena does not regret having surgery. "No, no, I don't regret having any of the surgeries," she informed us. However, she continued, "Now that I'm forty-four, I regret going so big." As pointed out earlier in this chapter, she believes the feminine beauty ideal has changed. While she once thought Pamela Anderson's body was in style, she now covets a lean athletic body with "normal" breasts. Moreover, hers have begun to sag. They are now a daily preoccupation. When asked how often she thinks about her breasts, she remarked, "About three to five times a day," continuing, "I [wish I] had gone 'normal.'"

Lena disclosed that body image struggles have plagued her throughout her lifetime. She was frank: "I have the worst body image, self-esteem." Her level of body dissatisfaction is high. She puts it at an eight or nine on a ten-point scale. It controls her everyday thinking and her daily actions. "I feel preoccupied about the way I look," she said honestly. Despite being single and open to the idea of meeting a new romantic partner, she said she has become so negative about her body that she "would die" before getting naked in front of someone. At the same time, she is clear that she passes no judgment on how others look: "I am so okay with what anybody else is." She commented that she would not have judged me as an interviewer whether I came with a hunched back or if I were a *Vogue* model.[21]

Lena attributes her intense body dissatisfaction and shame to her locale. "Orange County is the worst," she said candidly, adding that she lives in an "area where everybody has to look a certain way." This local obsession with looks comes with ongoing judgment: "Just living in this area, being around here, everybody is comparing everything. I think that's the biggest thing. . . . It's just like everybody is looking and judging around here." And they do not hold back: "People say mean things [to others] about the way they look."

She is immersed and trapped in what she deems an inescapable beauty culture. There is tremendous pressure to look a certain way, and criticism and low self-esteem accompany noncompliance. Her mom's normalization of cosmetic surgery is part of this. "Yeah, my parents [influenced my decision to have surgery] because my mom was up to it. She was like, 'If you want to go do it, do it. If you don't like the way it looks, fix it.'" Lena's fix-it mind-set is manifest in her ongoing beauty labor. She regularly uses nonsurgical cosmetic procedures such as Botox and Juvéderm.

Lena passionately believes that this beauty and fix-it-through-more-beauty-labor culture is "absolutely oppressive." During our conversation, she remarked that research funds used to advance cosmetic surgery should be directed to fund something more valuable, such as breast cancer research. She wept as she reflected on how cosmetic surgery negatively affects young girls and women:

[I think it is] absolutely oppressive. I think it's the worst thing in the world, and yet here I am. I think it just totally adds to the world's view that what you look like is so much more important than who you are, or what you have to give, or what you can do and be. I think people are, myself included, totally obsessed with, this is how a pretty woman looks, this is how a handsome man looks, this is how whatever looks. . . . I just think that, I think there should be a lot more education. . . . Girls need to be raised so much more caring about being smart. You know what I mean? It's sad. It's just sad. . . . I think there is way too much emphasis placed on [looks], and I know so many people who just suffer from it. I think it's very oppressive, and I think it sucks, because it's for an elite part of the population, but it's part of the population that the rest of the world sees. So you're sitting in the middle of the country, looking at the Grammys and going, "Oh my God, that's what I am supposed to look like."

The Grammy Awards took place in the Staples Center in Los Angeles a few weeks before our meeting. Among other cultural icons, Taylor Swift, Beyoncé, and Katy Perry were in the limelight. Their beautiful faces and bodies, Lena believes, set the standard for the rest of the country. She sobs when talking about how unrealistic beauty ideals send a message to girls and women that they should be valued more for their looks than their intellect. In her ideal world, this cultural logic would be reversed. However, despite her emotional plea and articulation that cosmetic surgery is the "worst thing in the world," she said that if money were not a consideration, she would undergo more surgeries, including a face-lift and buttock surgery. Her ongoing beauty labor—surgical or not—suggests a never-ending pursuit of body satisfaction and esteem.

Wishing She Embraced Her Unique Beauty

We met Carla when she was twenty-eight. She was working as a part-time program coordinator at a local public university while completing her college degree. At the time of her interview, she had been married for two years and had three young children. Carla had breast surgery at age twenty-four, which she had contemplated for about six years. She was a teenage mom, and after several years of breastfeeding, she felt "the overskin, it was just not nice. I didn't like it." She also said she suffered from "baby blues, like depression" and wanted to "do something extreme to feel better." However, her aunt persuaded her to hold off on surgery until she finished having children. So after delivering her third and decidedly last child, she booked a consultation with a cosmetic surgeon.

Carla went with the surgeon her mother-in-law and aunt had hired for their surgeries. The referral meant she was able to get a discount. She paid $400 down and put the remaining $3,200 balance on CareCredit. Her boyfriend (now spouse) was working full time. He ended up paying off the balance. Carla then paid him back. As recounted in Chapter 4, despite his financial assistance, Carla insisted she had surgery for herself, not him. "I don't want it to be connected to anybody but myself. Because I didn't like the way I looked. It wasn't what anybody else told me. It was what I felt."

In the days leading up to surgery, Carla was "really, really excited." She was not worried about the pain because her aunt and mother-in-law had assured her it was just a "little discomfort." This excitement soon dispelled when "they were doing all the markings on me, [and] that's when I started freaking out." She began to panic and said to her boyfriend, "I don't really think I want to do this, and I think I'm making a big missssstaaaake." According to Carla, he calmed her down, and she went through with surgery—a decision she questioned instantly afterward. This was her reaction upon seeing her altered breasts for the first time:

> I was so, like, freaked out because I . . . when I was doing the lines on me before the surgery I asked him for big C. . . . Then, um, when I saw them, they were huuuumooongous. Like, nothing like what I expected. No, I never expected them that big, and they were, like, way up, like, almost at my throat, you know. So I really got scared, like, I don't want to look like this.

Her surgeon reassured her that the swelling would eventually subside and her breasts would be smaller. She thought, "I hooooope, because this is really freaking me out. I was already picturing in my head, I'm going to have breast reduction one day soon! [*Laughs.*]"

Four years after her surgery, she is still wrestling with the size of her breasts. She felt her mother-in-law swayed her to "go a size or two bigger. So I kinda followed her advice, and I'm not happy." She maintains that she initially wanted a B or small C and was not even contemplating a large C or bigger. After surgery, she confronted her

surgeon: "I told him, 'I asked you for a C,'" to which he replied that
he needed to see what fit her, and in his view a D was "perfect" for
her. She suspects there was also confusion during her preoperative
consultation:

> My husband [then boyfriend], when we were doing the [preop-
> erative] checkup, he screamed something out like, "Order her
> a D!" And I think that stuck with him [the surgeon]. And he
> [the surgeon] said, "I thought you said a D, too. And you know
> it just fit you"—because I breastfed. I had room, I don't know
> [*laughs*]. [After surgery] he said that it fit perfect with me. He
> said they look beautiful. He said, you know, they're going to
> settle, you'll see. You'll get used to them. Okay. I dealt.

In Carla's view, her husband's joke to "order her a D" influenced the
surgeon's actions. She believes he did not honor her request made the
day of surgery—"I asked him for big C or a C." When asked if she is
upset with him, she said no. Rather, she is upset with herself. Echoing
Ana Marie's sentiment, she stated frankly, "I'm upset with myself for
not being clear on what I wanted."

We reported earlier that cosmetic surgery can lead to lifestyle
changes. For Carla, her disproportionately large breasts changed
how she exercises and sleeps, as well as the way she dresses. "I love
to run. I'm a runner," she said. Before surgery, she would often leave
the house and go for a run, sometimes even without a bra. But now,
she must "wear three sports bras or two good sports bras." And when
she does run, she says, "Most of the time I get a backache." She now
thinks twice about other activities such as hiking or biking. She said,
"It's more difficult; it's not the same anymore, [and] I get really bad
backaches afterwards." The surgery also affects how she sleeps. "I
love to sleep stomach down," she explained, but to avoid pain she
must sleep on her back or side. Additionally, because Carla believes
her breasts are noticeably large, she is "really careful" about how she
dresses. She is aware that she can "look really tacky or inappropriate."
One time at work her boss commented to all staff that they have to
"dress appropriately"—a message she believes was aimed at her. She
no longer wears V-neck shirts and admits to having a hard time find-

ing tops because she believes her breasts are disproportionately large for her 5'0", 126-pound body.

Despite these lifestyle adjustments, Carla says she does not regret having breast surgery. She only "regrets getting them the size [she] did." She plans to get a reduction when finances permit: "My ideal goal is in a few years either completely taking them off when I have the money or making them smaller. Way smaller!" She feels that at the time she had the surgery it was a reasonable decision because she was not happy and suffering from low self-esteem—a cognitive framing that enables her to reduce dissonance. "I think I did what I had to for my state of mind at that time. . . . Everything happens for a reason. I learned my lesson," Carla reflected. And with the fuller breasts she has gained "much more self-confidence." She strives to see the positive of surgery: "I looked like a little girl because I didn't have much breasts, but then with the breast [implants], I felt more like a woman. I was upset that they were so big, but at the same time I was like, 'Maybe this can be something good.'"

Her views of beauty have evolved, partly because of her experiences with cosmetic surgery, partly because of her ongoing college education, and partly because of her daughter. "I feel like, instead of changing ourselves, we need to change our perception of what beauty is [*pauses*] especially in California [*laughs*]. It is so hard!" She also feels that pursuing her college degree and being a sociology major have helped her better understand beauty culture and the role of social structures. She continued by discussing her daughter, who is a burn survivor:

Two years ago my daughter suffered from, um [*pauses*], an accident, and she is a burn survivor. So she is very, very scarred. She has burn scars. So that situation really, really changed my views on beauty, because, before, I feel like, you know, beauty looks a certain way, what I think most mainstream media, people believe beauty is. But after that, I feel like we all have our scars. We all have our stretch marks. We all have whatever it is we have. And that's what makes us beautiful. How different we all are, and we embrace that. And I feel like if I would continue to think the way I used to think, which is, you know, big boobs

and bottle-shaped model-looking-beautiful that's beautiful,
then I would be putting down my daughters. And that is just
horrible. You know, I need to teach them other ways. I need to
teach them the truth. . . . I feel like I was disgusted with the
way my breasts looked because they did not look like the girl in
the magazine. If I really embraced my uniqueness and I was in
love with myself, I feel like I would have been like, "So what!"
This is me, and this is what makes me beautiful.

Carla now redefines beauty as uniqueness. In hindsight she wishes
she had not been so fixated on cultural ideals of femininity and instead accepted what cultural norms deem flaws. She believes we all
have scars and stretch marks. Had she been more accepting of her
body, it is possible she would not have had surgery. She also believes
that if she continues to endorse the narrow definition of beauty found
in fashion magazines, then her daughters would not be beautiful—a
message she refuses to embrace. Nowadays she does not recommend
cosmetic surgery to others: "I would convince people not to do it."
Aside from corrective surgery, new surgeries are definitely off the
table for her. "No, never," she stated without hesitation.

When she finishes her college degree Carla hopes to continue
spreading a message of self-acceptance and self-love. During our interview, she opened up about having a tough time as a teenage mom
and having low self-esteem. She is passionate about helping others.
She has her sights set on becoming a high school counselor. "I still
feel like I have work to be done with myself, and I feel like that's going
to be an ongoing process," she said. "But I really want to positively
influence these young students."

Individual versus Cultural Change

Mainstream media stories about cosmetic surgery are often either
awe-inspiring success narratives or jaw-dropping tragedies. In reality, experiences of cosmetic surgery are neither. Sometimes women
are thrilled with their bodies immediately after surgery but voice
a very different opinion years later. Bodies, together with cultural
norms about the body, change, and women reinterpret surgical out-

comes throughout their lifetimes. These dynamic interpretations are made in consideration of ongoing boundary work in which women distance themselves from an abject surgical other. Over time, it is possible that a woman who once embodied the natural fake is left negotiating a body that is no longer surgically inconspicuous. She must then invoke physical and psychological strategies to manage a self and body that have come to resemble the surgical other. The specter of the surgical other always looms.

We witnessed this with four participants who have a complicated relationship with cosmetic surgery. Rebecca (discussed in Chapter 4) and Lena, who both belong to white, suburban, upper-middle-class social networks, struggled to escape what they condemn as an omnipotent and omnipresent beauty culture that makes unrealistic aesthetic demands of women. They struggled with their decision to go under the knife, conceding that they were caving to cultural pressures. Although first content with their enhanced body parts, disappointment eventually set in. Both articulated a desire to address disappointment by having future surgery. They were also open to having new forms of cosmetic surgery. In contrast, when faced with postoperative breasts they felt were conspicuous and unnaturally large for their bodies, both Ana Marie and Carla, who identify as Hispanic, downplayed their discontentment by redefining their personal conceptions of beauty. Both have now sworn off cosmetic surgery.

All four women, however, have something in common. They all desire a change in the detrimental beauty culture that feminist scholars have long claimed oppresses girls and women.[22] Yet all their responses, begot by disappointment, are individualized. Illustrating the power of social networks and underscoring the importance of social class, Rebecca and Lena say they will continue to partake in this beauty culture. Cosmetic surgery, it appears, has become a way of life. They are embedded in Southern California's beauty culture, and the solution to body dissatisfaction lies within it. Ana Marie and Carla opt to focus on self-acceptance and to redefine beauty on their own terms. In both sets of scenarios, the individualized solutions pose limited challenges to current cultural and social structures. The ubiquitous and powerful hegemonic discourses that prompted them to turn initially to cosmetic surgery thus remain firmly intact.

Resolving Paradoxes

Twenty-first-century women in America have made many strides compared with their foremothers. Women now compose nearly half the U.S. labor force, are more likely than men to be college educated, and hold leadership roles in business and government at record numbers.[1] Yet juxtaposed to these advances are a long list of inequalities, including pervasive wage disparity, rampant violence against women, and renewed threats to women's reproductive autonomy.[2] Moreover, nearly three decades after author and journalist Naomi Wolf wrote *The Beauty Myth*—a powerful and critical exposé of feminine beauty ideals[3]—these ideals continue to have negative health outcomes for women.[4] Women who chase the beauty myth, some feminist scholars maintain, are victims of patriarchy and capitalism.[5] They discipline their bodies through physically and emotionally harmful, as well as economically costly, body regimens and practices.[6] In this view, women who have cosmetic surgery bow to cultural pressures, and their ongoing attempts to embody hegemonic ideals, successful or not, reify these ideals in the long run.

At the same time, a makeover culture encourages women to draw on tools at their disposal to improve their lives.[7] Consequently, scholars like Kathy Davis maintain that women who undergo cosmetic surgery to address body dissatisfaction are merely taking control.[8] They use technological and medical advances, such as cosmetic surgery, to look and feel better. Within a neoliberal consumer marketplace, their decision can be interpreted as reasonable. They are postfeminist women with agency[9]—architects of their destinies acting in their own interests. Marketplace logics reward them for beauty compliance. This is because beauty is a status characteristic, and beauty capital translates into economic and social capital, seriously shaping life outcomes and social-psychological well-being.[10] Here, cosmetic surgery is empowerment.

The oppression-empowerment debate provides the theoretical backdrop of our research. It is in consideration of these competing perspectives, as well as the notion that the self is not fixed but dynamically reconstituted in light of social relations and structures,[11] that we seek to understand meanings about women's bodies. Within a beauty and makeover culture that emphasizes women's aesthetic transformation, one expects widespread body dissatisfaction. Yet women who address dissatisfaction through cosmetic surgery create a new set of problems. They choose a method that, despite claims of its cultural normalization and medicalization,[12] remains stigmatized. How do they address this paradox—these contradictory cultural discourses that place pressure on them to transform their bodies but stigmatize them for doing so?

We interviewed forty-six women from varied backgrounds who had different forms of cosmetic surgery to understand how they manage the stigma of a surgically altered body. In *Under the Knife*, we explore their motivations and views of stigma (Chapter 2), their pursuit and understanding of "natural" outcomes (Chapter 3), how they symbolically distance themselves from others (Chapter 4), and how they handle and negotiate surgery complications and disappointments (Chapter 5). In this closing chapter, we recap our empirical findings, attempt to make sense of them, and ask: Why does all this matter?

The Salience of Normative Femininity

Our participants' stories point to the overwhelming salience of gendered embodiment and "doing gender."[13] Participants admitted they were not immune to cultural pressures and said that cultural images are influential and create a desire to look feminine. Notably, none of the women we spoke with believed they could look, or even desired to look, like models in high-fashion magazines. Their verbal and facial expressions conveyed that this would be absurd. Rather, they aimed to enhance their appearance to align with mainstream constructs of femininity. This desire was evident across racial and ethnic lines, confirming the influence of a homogenizing hegemonic ideal.[14] Even when Latinas in our sample said that they felt cultural pressure from their ethnic communities to embody a Hispanic ideal, they felt that these ideals were consistent with a so-called American ideal—one that celebrates a taut and curvy body. Thus, at a time when cultural and structural barriers are slowly dismantling for women and norms about gender rigidity are relaxing—at least in terms of increased public awareness about gender and sexual fluidity—women from various racial and ethnic backgrounds still feel the weight of feminine beauty ideals. Their bodies continue to be a source of normative discontent.[15]

Relatedly, and confirming extant research on cosmetic surgery motivations,[16] participants had cosmetic surgery because they desired normalcy. They hoped to achieve normal everyday womanhood and "do gender" in everyday life. Cosmetic surgery enabled them to feel better about their bodies and blend in as feminine so they could engage in mundane activities with increased confidence, whether it was clothes shopping or going to the beach. It also allowed them to reap the rewards of normative femininity in dating and employment settings. They had cosmetic surgery, stressing that they did so on their own terms sans coercion, in the name of self-improvement. From their vantage point, they are simply good female citizens who advance themselves in a makeover culture. They are not oppressed but, rather, empowered agents whose motivations reflect a postfeminist outlook.

The Persistence of Cosmetic Surgery Stigma

The method our participants used to embody normative femininity has a long history. The historian Elizabeth Haiken notes that in 600 BC India a Hindu surgeon described what might be considered the first nose reconstruction.[17] Fast-forward two millennia. Today, in the same breath that women chat about CrossFit or the ketogenic diet, they might chat about Botox injections, dermal fillers, and cosmetic surgery. Aesthetic medical procedures are so pervasive in everyday discourses that some scholars surmise there is a new "aesthetic of artificiality."[18] This supposed normalization of cosmetic surgery[19] comes hand in hand with medicalization. When human conditions are defined as medical problems, medicine purports to hold the solution—for example, psychological or physiological intervention.[20] Medicalization also reduces the stigma associated with these conditions and normalizes medical solutions.[21] Nowadays, body image has come under the purview of medicine.[22] Thus, women today feel legitimated in their efforts to seek professional medical help to address body dissatisfaction, whether surgical or therapeutic.

Despite discourses of cultural normalization and medicalization, people who have cosmetic surgery are still statistical anomalies. Among the most common procedures that women have, only breast augmentations and tummy tucks have increased over the last two decades.[23] And in their lifetimes only a small percentage of U.S. adults (who are mostly white women) will go under the knife.[24] This infrequent resort may be connected to its negative image. Sure, it has become less taboo to talk about it, and mainstream media regularly covers it, but this does not mean it is stigma-free. The public continues to hold narrow perceptions of cosmetic surgeons,[25] and women who have surgery are criticized for psychological and aesthetic deficiencies. They are condemned for being and looking artificial.[26] Our interviews reinforce past research showing that the negative social judgment surrounding cosmetic surgery is not lost on those who have it.[27] Participants readily acknowledged the prevailing public sentiment that cosmetic surgery is unnecessary, a waste of money, indicative of superficiality and vanity, and evidence of personal failure—both a failure to change one's body through culturally acceptable means such as dieting and exercising and a failure to accept one's body as is.

Women's social location, however, shapes both their perceptions and experiences of stigma. Networks informed by geographic locale, class, race, and ethnicity can be a source of pressure to comply with beauty norms as well as an insulator to stigma for those who do have cosmetic surgery. For example, white participants situated in socioeconomically privileged social networks told us that cosmetic procedures were commonplace and nonchalantly discussed among friends and family members. Cosmetic surgery is so taken for granted that women who do not have surgery are sometimes labeled an "oddball." Additionally, these women feel inordinate pressure to live up to feminine beauty ideals. A keeping-up mentality, particularly in Southern California, meant that they were constantly engaging in body projects.

Ethnic communities can foster a similar mind-set. For example, despite mentioning that American ideals more or less align with Hispanic ideals, several Latinas in our sample felt compelled to keep up with Hispanic ideals—particularly the notion that Hispanic women should be well endowed. And our one Persian participant said that Persian culture patrols women's bodies, demanding perfection. In the end, the same networks and communities that exert pressure on women to achieve cultural perfection deem cosmetic surgery a legitimate panacea. The same oppressive beauty culture that places pressure on women to have surgery rewrites the cultural script, making cosmetic surgery a normative and less stigmatized solution.

It is not altogether surprising that cultural communities and social networks shape experiences of the body, as well as perceptions about beauty practices. The embracing of mainstream beauty ideals may make it more or less acceptable to have cosmetic surgery, and researchers have documented that the valuing of mainstream body ideals varies by, among other things, racial and ethnic background. For example, research shows more flexible conceptions of beauty in black communities.[28] Relatedly, some research shows that individuals from ethnic minority groups possess better body esteem and more positive body image than whites.[29] Some researchers speculate that this may result in a decreased need to enhance appearance. That is, more flexible conceptions of beauty and greater body satisfaction in some ethnic communities may translate into a decreased need to embody mainstream ideals via cosmetic surgery. A novel study examining ethnic differences in attitudes toward cosmetic surgery found that even after controlling for body appreciation, self-esteem, age, and body mass index, whites had higher acceptance of cosmetic surgery than ethnic minority groups.[30] These studies are consistent with the national demographic distribution of cosmetic surgery that is reflected in our sample; it is primarily white women who have it. These studies also show the importance of subcultures in shaping meaning making about body ideals and beauty practices.

Stigma Management

Even when social location and networks temper the stigma of cosmetic surgery, larger cultural discourses that stigmatize cosmetic surgery remain at work. And, as the classic work of the sociologist Erving Goffman tells us, stigma must be managed.[31] Social scientists have examined how people with different forms of stigma—from the stigma of HIV/AIDS to voluntary childlessness[32]—use strategies to minimize the negative repercussions of stigma and preserve a valued sense of self. These strategies come in many forms.[33] For example, research shows that "overweight" individuals employ deviance exemplars to manage a stigmatized identity[34] and passing techniques in the public sphere.[35] The elective nature of cosmetic surgery may intensify the need for stigma management. This is because research shows that when people believe a physical attribute is within a person's control, they are more likely to stigmatize this person. For example, people feel justified in openly criticizing someone who is obese when they believe that this person's obesity is caused by a lack of exercise. In contrast, if they believe that this person's obesity is caused by a glandular condition outside her control, this person is off limits for criticism.[36] Elective surgery clearly falls into this former category—within one's control.

Certainly, we are not the first to observe the exigencies of stigma management that cosmetic surgery begets. The sociologist Debra Gimlin claims that cosmetic surgery patients must "counter the charges of its inauthenticity."[37] She argues that women experience a "double bind"—while they are unhappy with their appearance, they must also defend their efforts to alter it.[38] The social researcher and analyst Preeta Saxena acknowledges that women who have breast surgery have "traded stigmas"—the stigma of breasts that do not live up to cultural norms for the stigma of breasts that are "not real" and come with negative stereotypes such as "bimbo."[39]

Both researchers report that cosmetic surgery patients use stigma management strategies. For example, Gimlin's early work examines narrative accounts—attempts to explain and justify deviant behavior and neutralize its negative meanings.[40] Much as our participants did, she shows how women account for cosmetic surgery as a financial investment that they worked hard for, as a needed change that allows them to take part in everyday life, and as a way of taking control of their bodies.[41] Some of Saxena's respondents, just as we saw with our participants' postfeminist rhetoric, resisted stigma by stressing that their decision was their own.[42] Other researchers report the use of justificational accounts, including self-worth accounts (e.g., surgery is done to feel better about oneself), interpersonal accounts (e.g., surgery is done so others would perceive them as normal), and material practices accounts (e.g., surgery is done to comply with prescriptions of femininity).[43] The limited research on men and cosmetic surgery reports that both patients' and surgeons' accounts of men's cosmetic surgery are gendered.[44] Specifically, patients and surgeons construct cosmetic surgery as "normal" and "natural" for women, whereas they construct men's concern for appearance as extrinsic. These accounts emphasize women's pursuit of aesthetic improvement as being intrinsic and essential to their nature. With men, surgery discourses center on instrumental purposes such as improving job prospects.

Similar to what we observed, Saxena and Gimlin find evidence for othering processes. Indeed, we borrow the term "surgical others" from Gimlin, a term she says includes "surgery junkies"[45] and women who have "gone too far" such as the so-called Cat Lady, Jocelyn Wildenstein.[46] Participants in her study distanced themselves from surgical others aesthetically when they maintained that these others have no understanding of natural feminine beauty and sacrifice a natural look for an artificial one. They drew socioeconomic boundaries by criticizing the surgical other for "excessive eagerness" to have surgery without "due consideration of its risks or costs"[47] and geographic boundaries by locating the surgical other elsewhere.[48] Specifically, Britons associated the surgical other with America, while some Americans associated it with Hollywood. Along the same lines, Saxena documents "stigma transference" and a "defensive othering" that occurs when "stigmatized individuals legitimate negative stereotypes and devalued identities by referring to 'others' to whom these stereotypes apply, but not to themselves."[49] For example, participants in her study voiced disgust for Beverly Hills moms and daughters who undergo cosmetic surgery to garner attention from men. These strategies enable women to distance themselves from discredited others.

Our research builds on these foundational studies. Although our findings replicate some themes arising from these earlier works, many of which focus on breast augmentation,[50] we flesh out these processes, extensively and systematically, by turning to in-depth interviews with women who had a range of surgical procedures. Unlike earlier work, our work focuses on participants' desire for and understanding of the natural, as well as on the processes that involve demarcating boundaries. Our examination of boundary work highlights the prominence of traditional gender discourses and our participants' construction of themselves as authentic, unique, and moral women. Moreover, because the interpretation of surgical outcomes fluctuates across the life course, the specter of the surgical other looms. There is always the possibility that one becomes the surgical other. The physical and psychological management strategies we document are thus crucial to women's continued identity management. The self is dynamic and, after surgery, continuously refashioned and managed. Ultimately, the strategies of passing, redefining, boundary work, and physical and psychological management enable women to preserve an authentic and gendered moral self—a self that, despite the articulation of postfeminist rhetoric, comports with traditional notions of femininity and virtue.

The Natural Fake as Cultural Honorific

Our interviews revealed a pervasive desire among our participants. They wanted natural surgical results. It was imperative that their postoperative bodies and body parts look "natural" and "not fake." Regardless of racial, ethnic, and class background and of procedure and body part, the majority of women we interviewed desired this outcome.

This desire is consistent with the literature on breast augmentation documenting that women who undergo cosmetic surgery desire a natural-looking body[51] and with writings by practitioners of aesthetic medicine who maintain that this is a goal of clients.[52] This desire also mirrors a common theme in the beauty and fashion industries. As some business scholars have observed, the natural look figures prominently in commercial fashion discourses.[53] A cursory look at a non-random sample of contemporary advertisements for beauty products and aesthetic medical procedures supports this. For example, one of Aveeno's marketing slogans is Naturally Beautiful Results, and a series of Aveeno advertisements with this slogan features the actress Jennifer Aniston wearing warm earth tones, relaxing in a light-colored setting, and smiling effortlessly at the viewer. Advertisements for lash and hair extensions place a similar emphasis on the natural. A JB Lashes advertisement promises a "natural look and feel," while a Secret Extensions advertisement claims its hair product will give you "thick, natural-looking volume and length in seconds!" A clinic for hair transplant and restoration emphasizes the company philosophy directly in the company name—Natural Transplants. There is even a brand of silicone gel implants called Natrelle, in all likelihood a clever marketing choice to evoke in consumers' imagination the sense that Natrelle implants resemble natural breasts.

Participants desired the natural fake. The natural fake allows its possessor to appear natural because the altered body part looks like it is either God-given (an inherent characteristic) or could have been achieved through nonsurgical means (such as diet or physical activity). In this way, it disguises its very own presence (hence, the centrality of inconspicuousness) and is natural. Yet it is also, rather paradoxically, an artificial achievement. First, it is made by trained surgeons who possess modern education and have the scientific know-how needed to perform surgery. An alteration by a surgeon's knowledgeable hand is undoubtedly a cultural intervention. Second, the natural fake mimics cultural norms. In actuality, there is really nothing natural about the natural fake. Certainly, the whole point of having surgery is to eliminate signs of nature, including any evidence of cultural body nonconformity that might accompany natural life course events such as aging and pregnancy (e.g., sagging and deflated breasts, loose skin, and unwanted flab). Via surgeons' hands, the natural fake encapsulates what is culturally celebrated and rewarded, socially and materially. Additionally, because it is a cultural achievement, it embodies quintessential ideals of femininity. One would expect nothing less than perfection from a technological intervention. Finally, achieving the natural fake requires significant unnatural intervention and investment. Prescriptions of normative femininity mandate the arduous and constant disciplining of the body.[54] They involve emotional, physical, and financial investment. Aniston's supposedly natural look prominently featured in Aveeno ads is anything but effortless and natural. It reportedly costs about $150,000 a year![55]

The marketing professors Craig J. Thompson and Diana L. Haytko have written about consumers' frequent use of *natural* when discussing fashion looks and icons. This term, they explain, is used as an honorific and associated with "positive meanings such as authenticity, an expression of timeless aesthetic principles, and freedom from fashion pressures." They suggest that references to the natural express a critique, whether implicit or explicit, of a look that is being displaced. They conclude, "The term 'natural' then functions as a mythic construct in the context of fashion discourse, that is, an amorphous ideal whose form is continuously reformulated in ways that sanction present-day standards." Thompson and Haytko further maintain that, compared with the new natural look, the displaced fashion is read by consumers as an "oppressive artificiality."[56] The natural fake operates in a similar manner. The *natural* of the natural fake is a symbolic term that captures something timeless, positive, and valued. This is in contrast to a body that is also technologically manipulated but embodies what is stigmatized and artificial. The *natural* here, however, is merely a placeholder, an honorific. In reality, the natural fake is a cultural embodiment that reflects what is acceptable and desirable at a given moment in time and space. While the natural fake today represents an inconspicuous, modest, and conservatively enhanced look, it could look very different a decade or two from now and may serve a very different function in relation to identity management.

In the meantime, women who embody the natural fake and its en vogue standards are able to pass, largely through concealment. Scholars have documented the use of cosmetic surgery to pass as normal[57] and have reported examples of racial and ethnic passing among individuals who use surgery to remove ethnic identifiers.[58] Similarly, the natural fake enables a woman to blend in with other women. By doing so, she limits the need to account for surgery in the first place. The natural fake therefore serves as a first line of defense against charges of artificiality and failure. Successful passing means avoiding the negative consequences of a stigmatized attribute and reaping the benefits of a nonstigmatized identity.

Redefining *Natural*

Given the prominence of the natural theme in participants' interviews, we asked them to explain what this term meant to them. They revealed that natural surgical outcomes conveyed either the appearance that they were born with the altered body part or that they achieved the altered body part without the surgeon's scalpel, such as through dieting and exercise. In both understandings, the desired results are inconspicuous and blend in with biological bodies. This inconspicuousness aligns with participants' motivation to be normal and achieve normative femininity. Their emphasis on conservative outcomes that are not extreme involved downplaying altered body parts as modest. Although participants insisted they would not lie about having surgery, they were delighted when others did not suspect they had, supposedly because their postoperative parts fit with and were appropriate for their bodies. At the end of the day, participants felt that surgery allows discreet feminine enhancement and restoration. All these characteristics are part of the larger package of the natural fake. Successful surgery is the inconspicuous natural fake.

Importantly, this framing of cosmetic surgery as modest enhancement enables participants to claim that their postoperative bodies are still natural. In their minds, they have not detoured so far from the God-given as to reach a point of artifice. Participants whose surgeries did not involve implants also said that their bodies could still be characterized as natural because they did not contain anything foreign requiring ongoing attention. Even participants who clung to an understanding of natural as unaltered by human influences insisted that, while they could no longer describe their bodies as natural, their bodies nevertheless *looked* natural. Regardless of the logic employed, these redefinitions serve as another line of defense against stigma. Women who go under the knife can assert that they are still natural or, at the very least, appear natural.

Evidence that women covet the natural fake contradicts research, albeit limited, showing that women want visibly fake breasts. The sociologist Jacqueline Sanchez Taylor found in her interviews with white working-class British women that they had no feelings of embarrassment or unease about having artificial breasts.[59] Instead, their surgically altered breasts marked them as economically successful and modern. Gimlin discovered something similar in her research with women who had breast augmentation. A handful of women she interviewed exhibited little preoccupation with "naturalness." Rather, they desired "voluptuous" and "fake-looking" breasts.[60] Both researchers argue that such breasts display women's ability to invest large financial resources in the body. That is, it is a form of conspicuous consumption[61] and provides a "symbolic link to the lifestyle practices of the successful, rich and famous."[62] For these outliers, fake breasts express class assumptions.[63]

The socioeconomic status of our participants might account for the predominance of participants' desire for the natural fake and a rejection of this fake-looking aesthetic. Only a handful of our participants reported personal incomes around or below poverty level,[64] and those who did were likely at this level in part because they were in school at the time of their interviews. The large number of middle- and upper-middle-class participants in our sample may suggest little need to display this type of class identity work. However, this form of conspicuous consumption, with its emphasis on showy body parts and evocations of a nouveau riche lifestyle, is likely unappealing to our participants because it runs counter to the type of boundary work that surfaced in their accounts of cosmetic surgery.

Boundary Work

Boundary work was coined by Thomas Gieryn, a sociologist who used the term to discuss scientists' efforts to distinguish their work from nonscientists. In a 1983 article published in the flagship journal of the American Sociological Association, *American Sociological Review,* Gieryn describes how scientists attribute certain characteristics to the institution of science for the purpose of creating a social boundary that distinguishes science from other nonscientific intellectual and professional activities.[65] These rhetorical practices protect professional autonomy and establish credibility and epistemic authority. Boundary work is thus about symbolic boundaries—lines that include some people, groups, and things at the exclusion of others.[66]

Since Gieryn's groundbreaking conception of the term, contemporary empirical research on boundaries continues to stress delineation processes to understand "self-definitions of ordinary people and in a range of contexts beyond science." The Harvard sociologist Michèle Lamont and her colleagues note that these studies include the work of social psychologists on segmentation—us versus them—and work by sociologists on how "boundary work is accomplished," specifically the typification systems and inferences concerning similarities and differences that groups use to define who they are.[67]

In the cosmetic surgery realm, women engage in boundary work to show who they are (us) and who they are not (them). This boundary work is first and foremost evident in participants' pursuit of the natural fake. Their exaltation of this construct accompanied condemnation of its antithesis—surgically altered body parts they deemed fake and artificial looking. They framed their surgeries as aesthetically pleasing and "obvious" surgeries as "unnatural" and "fake" aesthetic abominations.

Although the majority of participants said that cosmetic surgery was not a requirement for life success, they exhibited another form of boundary work when they framed their surgeries as necessary. Here they turned the cosmetic surgery paradox on its head. A cultural beauty hierarchy that rewards self-improvement and beauty compliance makes surgery necessary if women are to be successful female subjects. When beauty is mandated for women and a woman has small breasts or a crooked nose, there is little she can do but have surgery. As one participant put it, "Exercise is not going to fix my breasts ever!" Even participants who had procedures involving fat removal, which hegemonic cultural discourses frame as cheating, said they did everything they could to get rid of saddlebags and stomach fat before consulting a surgeon. Despite ongoing efforts through dietary restrictions and exercise, they were not able to change these body parts, rendering surgery necessary.

While our participants are by no means experiencing the type of social death the sociologist Heather Laine Talley writes about in her study of the facially disfigured, her work nevertheless encourages us to rethink the notion that aesthetic surgeries are not lifesaving and by extension necessary.[68] As she underscores, cultural hierarchies enforce narrow conceptions of aesthetic acceptability and discriminate against those who do not conform to hegemonic body ideals. In light of the real social, economic, and psychological consequences of beauty nonconformity, it is reasonable for women to invoke the logic of necessity to account for their surgeries. Furthermore, as the law professor Deborah Rhode asserts, physical characteristics can be conceptualized along a continuum.[69] Traits deemed immutable (such as skin color and height) are on one end of this continuum, and traits deemed mutable (such as hair color and body weight) are at the other. Discrimination against the former traits, Rhode argues, has come to be regarded as unjustified and even illegal because they are typically unchangeable and outside a person's control. In contrast, because the latter traits supposedly stem from personal choices, they are not legally protected. On top of that, they are open to social scrutiny. It thus makes sense for participants to account for their body parts as immutable without cosmetic surgery. Such framing serves as a potential shield to social criticism—stigma is unwarranted and unacceptable because that specific body part is beyond their control.

There is, however, some notable variation in participants' understanding of what constitutes necessary. When they say surgery is necessary, this does not mean they are saying *all* cosmetic surgery is. Reflecting dominant ideologies about body modification, dieting, and weight loss[70] that reflect an antifat bias,[71] some participants who had breast or nose surgery explicitly said they would not have procedures involving fat removal. By maintaining this position, they passed judgment on people who have, for example, liposuction. In their opinion, these types of surgeries are not needed because the body can be sculpted through behavioral changes alone. They believe this despite substantial evidence to the contrary—for example, that dieting is generally ineffective.[72]

Variations in participants' conceptualization of *necessary* surgery illustrate the nuances of boundary work and how various forms of surgeries can be pitted against one another. Another example of this surfaced when participants whose surgeries did not involve implants maintained that their postoperative bodies were still natural, contra, as they pointed out, surgical others who have foreign objects in their bodies. In this way, boundary work is about limits of acceptability in which even those in the us camp may not always agree. The sociologist Ranita Ray's research on economically marginalized young black and Latina women is instructive here.[73] She observes that these young women create "identities of distance." By establishing themselves as independent, self-reliant, and ambitious, they distance themselves from risk narratives of stigmatized teen parenthood. However, Ray claims that in the process of othering those whom they see as pregnancy risks, they create a moral self that reinforces the notion of "early parenthood in marginalized communities as inherently problematic."[74] That is, boundary work can further entrench the stigma associated with the social phenomenon at hand. In a similar manner, participants' boundary work (and especially these layers of boundary work) can reinforce the stigma associated with cosmetic surgery, continuing to frame it as problematic and in need of justification.

Participants also distinguished their "good" surgeries from "bad" ones. Good surgeries begin with competent board-certified surgeons who are not hacks. They turned to the best they could afford, finding surgeons through word of mouth and internet search engines. Before and after pictures on surgeons' websites helped them evaluate whether a surgeon could deliver the natural fake. Participants' vision of a clean, modern surgeon's office in the United States contrasts with a negative stereotype of a practitioner in the global south who, in their minds, might not even be licensed. Such a distinction process clearly has classist and ethnocentric undertones yet is not entirely unexpected given select media coverage of cosmetic surgery cases gone awry in South America. For example, the arrest of Brazilian plastic surgeon Denis Furtado, who performed buttock enhancement surgery in his home, received international media attention.[75] At the same time, cues about a surgeon's competence are sometimes based on positive (and similarly narrow) stereotypes. For example, the model minority stereotype[76] of an Asian surgeon swayed at least one participant who was convinced his ethnicity meant he would pay more attention to detail—a belief consistent with research that documents clients' racial biases against Asian beauty service workers.[77]

Women who have cosmetic surgery also see themselves as good patients. They are psychologically sound and do not have deep psychological issues. Sure, women can turn to cosmetic surgery to increase confidence and self-esteem, but their starting point is not so low as to merit the label of psychological pathology. Once again, postfeminist rhetoric comes to the fore; good patients have reasonable expectations and are motivated by self-improvement—whether of material well-being that betters one's life situation, psychological well-being that addresses the psyche, or physical well-being that improves lifestyle and health. Much as weight loss surgery can serve as a point of rebirth,[78] some participants said they used cosmetic surgery to motivate a healthier lifestyle. They slammed celebrities who have multiple surgeries, and they said that they are not cosmetic surgery "junkies." Their words mirror cultural discourses that praise them for embarking on body projects. As one participant explained, women who have cosmetic surgery are "more in touch" with themselves because they take steps to address dissatisfaction and improve themselves.

Thus, time and time again, participants framed their decision to have cosmetic surgery through a postfeminist lens. They are not oppressed victims but, rather, reasonable women of sound mind who are motivated to improve their lives. In consultations, surgeons too confirmed their views of them as good patients, thereby strengthening their boundary work. Surgeons informed them that they operated only on patients, like them, who have reasonable standards and are mentally healthy. As Gimlin observes in her research, surgeons vet patients for mental stability and are collaborators in boundary work.[79] This vetting is a form of boundary work that surgeons perform to convey the message that they are not just stereotypical "boob job surgeons," flashy and trying to make a fast buck.[80]

Interestingly, white participants' boundary work often involved invoking a surgical other who is white and female.[81] This contrasts the typical construction of the other and otherness. The other is a cultural category that represents a binary opposite; the categories of the binary are, as the philosopher Simone de Beauvoir argues, uniquely defined in relation to one another.[82] Thus, when thinking about and discussing cosmetic surgery, these women distance themselves from an undesirable standard that they can align with in terms of gender and race but that they nevertheless deem lacking. For example, white participants dismissed Barbie as bland, disparaged celebrities such as Pamela Anderson for looking artificial, and condemned their own daughters for getting breasts that were "too big." The "beach bunnies" and "river rats" white California participants alluded to are presumably white. The quintessential pinup of the California beach bunny depicts a tall, thin, hourglass-figure white woman in her early twenties with long flowing blonde hair. She displays ample cleavage in her bikini as she poses seductively by the Pacific Ocean.

In contrast, there appears to be greater variation in the racial and ethnic referent invoked by the women of color in our sample. For example, a number of Hispanic and Asian participants referenced Barbie (again, as symbolic of the cookie-cutter fake and thus to be avoided). And when discussing alienation, African American participants mentioned cultural figures such as Nicki Minaj and Kim Kardashian.[83] Although the latter is white, she can be culturally coded as nonwhite. Hence, at the same time that the surgical other is not a racial and ethnic other for white women, the surgical other can be white or nonwhite for racial and ethnic minority women.

This flexibility in how women of color discuss the surgical other suggests evidence for the influence of white cultural beauty ideals. Whether consciously or not, participants illustrate that white ideals have symbolic sway, at least in their articulations of these matters. This is consistent with the lack of racial and ethnic diversity in mainstream media depictions. Scholars continue to show the pervasiveness of Eurocentric beauty standards in mainstream media and its detrimental effects on girls and women of color.[84] Only in the last few years has Mattel introduced the Fashionistas line of Barbies with diverse skin tones, hair types, and eye shapes.[85] It is possible that as cultural images become more diverse, women of color will come to define the self, as well as the surgical other, more exclusively along racial and ethnic lines, and white women will begin to broaden their cultural conceptions.

Identity Work, Postfeminism, and the Madonna-Whore Dichotomy

Boundary work is identity work.[86] Women who have cosmetic surgery say they are this and not that to preserve an identity that is congruent with how they see themselves. They desire to project a certain sense of self to the world. Despite the physical changes brought about by surgery, women who have cosmetic surgery reassure themselves and the people around them that they remain true to themselves. They are reasonable and empowered women who embark on projects of self-improvement and are still good mothers, workers, students—

only, version 2.0 or 3.0. Unlike surgical others whose surgeries they denigrate as dramatic and obvious, participants embody the natural fake. In doing so, they can say that they still look like themselves and, by extension, are still themselves.

Participants stressed preserving the face, a part of the body that has special social and personal significance. As Talley explains, the face is a "powerful biosocial resource" that conveys information about our age, race, ethnicity, gender, and social class, and facial appearance affects our life chances and opportunities.[87] Moreover, she argues that the face is a mechanism for communicating "core facets of our identities" and "is capable of mediating human subjectivity and public personhood."[88] Precisely because our face is tied to our social identity, participants expressed caution about altering it and condemned reality television contestants whose extreme makeovers left them virtually unrecognizable. Participants who had face-lifts reassured themselves after surgery that they could still recognize themselves in the mirror. The natural fake enables this. They just look like a younger or refreshed version of themselves, they reasoned. The significance of the face is likely why some participants were leery about the use of facial injections such as Botox or going overboard with facial fillers.

An emphasis on retaining an authentic self comes hand in hand with projecting a unique and moral self. Despite the homogenizing effects of cosmetic surgery,[89] participants insisted that surgery did not make them appear generic. Furthermore, they insisted that this type of body project should not signify to the world that they are preoccupied with beauty and sexuality. Participants actively distanced themselves from "those women"—"river rats" and "beach bunnies" who are "all boobs." The political theorist Iris Marion Young has written about how breasts are sexual signifiers,[90] and participants who had breast surgery were especially concerned others would code them as hypersexual. They resented the association of breast surgery with porn stars and downplayed the size of their breast implants. A number of women even said they dressed more modestly after surgery to avoid drawing attention to their bodies in the workplace or in social engagements. Large breasts are undeniably an exalted form of feminine sex appeal, yet participants feel compelled to cover up their surgically modified breasts to display modesty.

There is considerable irony to this type of boundary-cum-identity work. Cosmetic surgery is a financial investment with physical, emotional, and social costs. Because it is associated with some attributes that are not exactly praiseworthy (e.g., frivolity, superficiality, and vanity) participants strive to embody the natural fake—an inconspicuous enhancement—and do cognitive work to define their postoperative bodies as natural or natural appearing. They also distance themselves from what they see as problematic aspects of the practice itself. In their accounts of surgery, they employ postfeminist empowerment language. They are women with agency who capitalize on available resources in the name of self-advancement.

However, there is a key difference between them and their postfeminist media counterparts. While Beyoncé is an active sexual subject who reveals quite a bit of her body in public—whether in her concerts, red carpet appearances, music videos, or social media communications—it appears that she does so with little reservation and concern about negative social repercussions. In fact, she profits generously from these public displays. In contrast, this sexual exhibition and liberation is not manifest in the lives of most everyday women. Instead, the everyday woman must practically and safely navigate precarious social settings and relationships—workplaces, school environments, family, sports and recreational spaces, dating, and more—where her sexuality is policed. We live in a rape culture where rape shield laws that are supposed to protect women from judgments about her displays of sexuality fail to serve their purpose.[91] Victim blaming and the sexual objectification of women are everyday facts of life.[92] Slut shaming is commonplace, online and off.[93] Physical and sexual violence against women, along with sexual harassment and stalking, are rampant.[94] Women are constantly judged for the way they look and how they behave. There are few safe spaces.

An example of the pervasive social control of women was brought to light when girls at a high school in Maryland discovered a list made by their male counterparts who ranked them by physical appearance.[95] This sexist practice is not novel given the history of the popular social networking service Facebook and its origins as FaceMash—a hot-or-not game that ranked female Harvard classmates' attractiveness.[96] At Rowan University, the university's athletic department moved the women's track-and-field practice to a local high school because the head football coach felt that women athletes running on the track in sports bras were "distracting" his male players.[97] On another campus, in a letter to the editor of the University of Notre Dame student newspaper, a Catholic mother chastised female students for wearing leggings, writing, "Leggings are so naked, so form fitting, so exposing. Could you think of the mothers of sons the next time you go shopping and consider choosing jeans instead?"[98] These are only a few examples of the ways women's bodies are policed in what is ostensibly a postfeminist society in which women's equality has been achieved and gender injustice is a thing of the past.

Thus, women who have cosmetic surgery effectively do normative femininity—a femininity that does not involve overly sexual displays of their body. Entrenched sexual scripts[99]—the social conventions that dictate sexual behaviors and serve as guides for people to interpret, as well as act in, sexual situations—reinforce this.[100] Heterosexual scripts, in particular, prioritize boys' and men's sexual desire and approve men as initiators. In contrast, these scripts construct women as passive and careful gatekeepers.[101] While he is expected to actively fulfill his sexual needs, she is expected to please him and wait on his actions. The developmental psychology professor Janna Kim and her colleagues capture well the essence of women's roles in these scripts when they write, "The Heterosexual Script compels girls/women to deny or devaluate their own sexual desire, to seek to please boys/men, to 'wish and wait,' to be chosen, and to trade their own sexuality as a commodity."[102] In short, sexual scripts limit women's sexual agency,[103] compelling them to tame and suppress their sexual self-expression.

At the core of women's postoperative identity work is thus the Madonna-whore dichotomy. This dichotomy presents polarized perceptions of women as either a Madonna (chaste and pure) or as a whore (promiscuous and seductive).[104] Like sexual scripts theory, this dichotomy works to limit women's sexual freedom.[105] Women who have cosmetic surgery are trapped in a Catch-22. Cosmetic surgery helps them improve their lives—to feel good, succeed in the workplace, find romantic partners, and so on—but because narrow sexual scripts and patriarchal structures result in the patrolling of their bodies, they must not flaunt their enhanced bodies. Consequently, their accounts emphasize the embodiment of the emblematic Madonna and a distancing from the symbolic whore.

Managing Disappointment and the Specter
of the Surgical Other

Research shows that cosmetic surgery patients are typically satisfied with surgical outcomes,[106] and this was evident in our sample. Participants were thrilled that surgery resulted in a more harmonious relationship with their bodies. They felt good about and motivated by their bodies. But alongside this general affirmation of cosmetic surgery were also stories about complications, struggles, and disappointments. We felt compelled to share these stories because, as a journalist writing for the *Atlantic* points out, we live in a "glib culture" that downplays the seriousness of cosmetic surgery, particularly the health problems that can accompany breast implants.[107]

Participants experienced a range of physical side effects, including infection, loss of sensation, erratic itching sensations, and scarring. With breast implants, they reported hardening, rupturing, wrinkling, and sloshing. Aesthetic disappointments centered on unevenness or a lack of noticeable change, which participants discussed in light of the financial, emotional, and physical drain that they felt accompanied surgery. For a handful of participants, with surgery also came some unexpected lifestyle changes, including lingering pain and changes in how they exercised and slept.

Sometimes disappointment set in years later. Large conspicuous breasts once in style were reinterpreted decades later as tacky. There were stories about perky and taut breasts succumbing to gravity. With time, participants' venerated natural fakes transformed into conspicuous aesthetic deviations that alarmingly resembled characteristics of the imaginary surgical other. These changes potentially trigger the need for further negotiations of the self, sometimes prompting additional surgery. Indeed, body image is a dynamic construct and, as sociocultural context changes, women encounter new experiences and reinterpret old experiences.[108]

To address physical complications and aesthetic disappointments, participants turned to physical management strategies, some of which have been reported by other researchers studying physical-appearance stigma.[109] For participants whose finances permitted, the simplest solution was to fix the problem by turning to medical experts—a strategy that is clearly classed (and by extension raced), because corrective surgery is not free. Participants also concealed problematic body parts (using clothing and makeup creams) and redirected attention from them (by playing up other aspects of their appearance and downplaying altered parts). Psychological management techniques, such as reasoning that results are never perfect, enabled a positive cognitive reframing so that the decision to have surgery did not lead to psychological anguish or long-term regret.

Finally, to expose the diverse meanings and experiences that come with cosmetic surgery, we shared the stories of four participants who exhibited a fraught relationship with cosmetic surgery. Each of these four women came to resemble select aspects of the surgical other—whether through their financial struggle, emotional struggle, or both. Their stories bring to light the resounding reality that cosmetic surgery is not always a cakewalk, while illuminating the role class, race and ethnicity, and geographic locale play in meaning making. We witnessed how difficult it was for two white participants who condemned cosmetic surgery as oppressive to escape their upper-middle-class suburban social networks. For them, cosmetic surgery is the problem, but it is also paradoxically the solution. We also witnessed how socioeconomic disadvantage put the fix-it approach out of reach for two Latina participants. Both could not afford to have corrective surgery. The two eventually channeled their postoperative disappointments into an appreciation for their bodies and selves. They vowed to embrace their unique beauty. Despite these very different life paths, these case studies show that women who have cosmetic surgery can still come to question the role it plays in their lives. Their challenges to the practice, however, are limited. They all resort to individualized solutions—either having more cosmetic surgery or turning to self-love. In doing so, they fail to shake the foundations of the powerful beauty discourses that foster women's body dissatisfaction and led them to cosmetic surgery in the first place.

Limitations and Future Directions

Faced with the cosmetic surgery paradox, women use various strategies to account for their surgeries, neutralize stigma associated with this type of beauty work, and manage physical and psychological challenges across the life course. Their strategies permit the preservation of a gendered moral self that, contra postfeminist rhetoric, aligns with traditional notions of femininity. Our through line thus emphasizes normative femininity. Yet our strictly U.S. female sample with a heteronormative and cisgender bias leaves plenty of room for further investigation of cosmetic surgery among men and people who identify as LGBTQ, gender fluid, or gender nonconformists, along with the meaning of cosmetic surgery at the intersections of these and other status characteristics (such as race, ethnicity, and disability). Do the natural fake and understandings of the natural, as well as identity and boundary work, translate to other populations, including those in other countries? Moreover, how do they apply to nonsurgical cosmetic practices and other beauty work practices—such as hair extensions, tanning, and artificial nails and lashes—which may also have natural implications? And while none of the women we interviewed were in the sex industry, examining the meanings of cosmetic surgery among sex workers would be an important line of future inquiry, particularly in consideration of our central claim that modern cosmetic surgery involves traditional displays of women's sexuality.

Researchers should continue to study racial and ethnic variations in understandings of the natural fake, boundary work, and identity work. While we pointed out raced, classed, and gendered dynamics that surfaced in our data, in the assertion of an authentic moral self there was a remarkable absence of racial and ethnic talk in participants' stories. Participants seemed more concerned with retaining a good feminine self than asserting a racial or ethnic identity. Their focus on gender normativity may be because no participant in our sample had racialized surgery. Consequently, their surgeries posed little threat to their racial and ethnic identities, perhaps quelling any need to reaffirm this aspect of the self.

However, cultural analysts have shown that light skin for women is associated with modesty, purity, and virtue, while dark skin is associated with sexual suggestiveness.[110] Researchers have also found that visual media sexually objectify and associate black women with animal imagery to a greater extent than white women.[111] Additionally, the sociologist Maxine Leeds Craig's research illustrates that young African American women have a complex and even contradictory understanding of beauty.[112] For example, they describe beauty as natural and defend the beauty of dark skin or natural hair at the same time that they equate (short) natural hair with neglect, failure at self-care, and even a desire to be a boy. They also reject extremes of femininity, such as false lashes, which they associate with artificiality, fakeness, and "acting white."[113] While cautioning that the dichotomy between white as artificial and black as authentic is simplistic, Craig's research points to how race is used to delineate boundaries of acceptability. All these observations potentially complicate, especially for women of color with darker skin, our argument about the natural fake and the postoperative modest self. We encourage others to explore further identity negotiation strategies along racial and ethnic lines, including those involving racialized cosmetic surgery.

In our conversations we also picked up on participants' use of what might be referred to as disembodied language. When describing their breasts, some participants used terms such as "these," "them," or "the girls." This language of alienation suggests a distancing and a more fractured self than the identity work we present here suggests. Whether and how identity work helps preserve a coherent and healthy postoperative self over time merits longitudinal investigation. Finally, while all our participants strove for normative femininity, even within accommodating practices, there can be resistance.[114] Can these accounts and negotiations of the self be retooled to exhibit embodied resistance? What is the role of social activism, such as the body positivity movement and the Health at Every Size movement,[115] in how women come to understand their aesthetic surgical practices and their dynamic sense of self? Furthermore, what is the role of these movements in removing the lingering stigma associated with cosmetic surgery?

Challenging Cultural Structures

Women are put in a no-win situation if their natural bodies and faces do not meet cultural expectations of feminine beauty because some body parts (like noses and breasts) cannot be changed (or at least not in ways that are culturally exalted) without surgery; accepted remedies to change seemingly mutable body parts, such as dieting, often fail;[116] and stigma still accompanies the extreme solution of going under the knife. Thus, women, who are socially encouraged and expected to chase the beauty myth, must either accept the repercussions of failing to live up to feminine beauty ideals or deal with the medical risks, as well as the psychological and social consequences, of having cosmetic surgery. Their out—which requires boundary work and identity work—is to obtain the natural fake. The natural fake allows them to pass as surgically unaltered while, in their minds, more closely living up to gendered appearance norms. Yet there is no guarantee that they will be more satisfied with their surgically altered bodies, especially as the interpretation of surgical outcomes fluctuates across the life course and the specter of becoming the surgical other always looms. Physical and psychological management, as well as management of the self, become a dynamic lifelong process.

While the *availability* of the natural fake is viewed by many women as empowering, the identity work that ensues involves women's ongoing self-policing and the assertion of a moral and modest self that reinforces traditional notions of feminine virtue. Moreover, it is born out of oppressive beauty ideals that ultimately harm women by continuing to define physical appearance as the centerpiece of womanhood. As activists and scholars before us have argued, there is a pressing need to redefine femininity and dethrone beauty as the defining quality of womanhood. We hope our work contributes to this process by shining a light on this cultural paradox and furthering the conversation about changing norms of femininity.

Appendix

Participants' Pseudonyms, Demographics, and Surgeries

Name	Age	Occupation/industry	Education	Marital status	Number of children	Race/ethnicity	Annual personal income	Surgeries	Surgery location
Allison	50	Administrative assistant	Some college	Divorced, widowed	3	White	$40,000 to $59,999	Breast augmentation	United States
Ana Marie	27	College student and part-time waitress	Bachelor's degree in progress	Married	1	Hispanic	Less than $19,999	Breast augmentation	United States
Ashley	24	Sales representative	Bachelor's degree	Single	0	Hispanic	$40,000 to $59,999	Breast augmentation	United States
Barbara	58	Media buyer	Some college	Married	1	White	$80,000 to $99,999	Trunk lift	United States
Caitlin	31	Stay-at-home mom and part-time substitute teacher	Master's degree in progress	Married	1	White	$60,000 to $79,999	Breast augmentation	United States
Carla	28	College student and part-time program coordinator	Bachelor's degree in progress	Married	3	Hispanic	Less than $19,999	Breast augmentation	United States
Casey	40	Unemployed, previously a technology specialist	Bachelor's degree	Married	0	White	$60,000 to $79,999	Breast reduction, liposuction	United States
Charlize	44	Real estate	Bachelor's degree	Divorced	1	White	$80,000 to $99,999	Breast augmentation (thrice)	United States
Chloe	29	Wedding consultant	Bachelor's degree	Married	0	Hispanic	$40,000 to $59,999	Thigh tuck	United States
Claronette	59	College (work study) student	Bachelor's degree in progress	Divorced	3	Black	$20,000 to $39,999	Tummy tuck	United States

Name	Age	Occupation	Education	Marital status	Children	Ethnicity	Income	Procedure	Country
Darla	27	College student and part-time personal assistant	Bachelor's degree in progress	Single	0	Hispanic	$20,000 to $39,999	Rhinoplasty	United States
Elaina	42	Stay-at-home mom and college student	Bachelor's degree in progress	Married	5	Hispanic	Less than $19,999	Rhinoplasty, ear surgery	Mexico
Grace	27	Staff associate	Bachelor's degree	Married	0	White	$60,000 to $79,999	Breast augmentation	United States
Hanna	21	College student and part-time waitress	Bachelor's degree in progress	Single	0	White	Less than $19,999	Breast augmentation, rhinoplasty	United States
Hazel	42	Personal trainer and nutrition counselor	Some college	Single	0	White	$20,000 to $39,999	Rhinoplasty (thrice), breast augmentation	United States
Heather	38	Teacher	Master's degree	Divorced	0	White	$60,000 to $79,999	Breast augmentation (twice)	United States
Janet	64	Media buyer	Bachelor's degree	Divorced	0	White	$60,000 to $79,999	Face-lift (twice), tummy tuck, breast augmentation	United States
Jasmine	24	Assistant restaurant manager and part-time college student	Bachelor's degree in progress	Single	0	White	$20,000 to $39,999	Breast augmentation, full body lift, liposuction	United States
Jenna	47	Office manager	Bachelor's degree	Single	0	White	$60,000 to $79,999	Rhinoplasty	United States
Jessica	68	Retired teacher	Bachelor's degree	Widowed, remarried	2	White	Not reported	Breast augmentation (twice)	United States
Kali	23	College student and part-time retail sales	Bachelor's degree in progress	Single	0	East Asian	$20,000 to $39,999	Tummy tuck	United States

(continued)

Name	Age	Occupation/industry	Education	Marital status	Number of children	Race/ethnicity	Annual personal income	Surgeries	Surgery location
Kaylee	20	College student	Bachelor's degree in progress	Single	0	Hispanic	Less than $19,999	Breast augmentation	United States
Kerrie	28	College student and part-time data entry clerk	Bachelor's degree in progress	Single	0	Asian	$60,000 to $79,999	Breast augmentation	United States
Kristen	24	Retail sales	Some college	Single	1	Black	$20,000 to $39,999	Breast augmentation, tummy tuck, liposuction	United States
Lacy	22	College student and part-time museum worker	Bachelor's degree in progress	Single	0	White	Less than $19,999	Liposuction	United States
Lavanna	32	Teacher	Master's degree in progress	Divorced	3	Black	$40,000 to $59,999	Tummy tuck	United States
Leanne	54	School counselor	Master's degree	Divorced	1	White	$120,000 to $139,999	Breast augmentation (twice)	United States
Leila	41	Correctional officer	Some college	Divorced	3	Black	$20,000 to $39,999	Breast reduction	United States
Lena	44	Stay-at-home mom	Master's degree	Divorced	2	White	$60,000 to $79,999	Rhinoplasty, breast augmentation (twice)	United States
Lily	28	Dentist	Professional degree	Engaged	0	White	$80,000 to $99,999	Rhinoplasty	United States

Name	Age	Occupation	Education	Marital status	Children	Race/Ethnicity	Income	Procedure	Country
Linda	57	Personal assistant and chef	Some college, professional certification	Single	0	Hispanic	$60,000 to $79,999	Rhinoplasty	United States
Lorna	33	Teacher	Bachelor's degree	Married	0	White	$40,000 to $59,999	Jaw surgery	United States
Marianne	54	Vice president, banking	Bachelor's degree	Divorced	0	White	$180,000 or more	Rhinoplasty, liposuction, breast augmentation, partial face-lift	United States
Martha	67	Retired interior designer	Bachelor's degree	Widowed	2	White	$120,000 to $139,999	Face-lift, tummy tuck, liposuction, body lift	United States
Nadine	62	Computer graphics design	Bachelor's degree	Divorced	2	White	$40,000 to $59,999	Liposuction (twice)	United States
Parvina	35	Medical resident	Professional degree	Single	0	Middle Eastern	Less than $19,999	Rhinoplasty	Iran
Penelope	61	Financial butler	Some college	Divorced	1	White	$180,000 or more	Breast augmentation, eyelid surgery, liposuction, face-lift	United States
Rebecca	40	Self-employed	Some college	Divorced	1	White	$20,000 to $39,999	Rhinoplasty (multiple), breast augmentation	United States
Reese	30	Small-business owner and part-time fast-food worker	Bachelor's degree	Single	0	White	$40,000 to $59,999	Breast augmentation	United States

(continued)

Name	Age	Occupation/industry	Education	Marital status	Number of children	Race/ethnicity	Annual personal income	Surgeries	Surgery location
Robin	38	Unemployed, previously a business analyst	Bachelor's degree	Divorced	3	White	$80,000 to $99,999	Tummy tuck	United States
Roxanne	50	Software consultant	Bachelor's degree	Divorced	2	White	$100,000 to $119,999	Breast augmentation	United States
Sarah	38	College student and small-business owner	Bachelor's degree in progress	Engaged	1	White	$60,000 to $79,999	Breast augmentation	United States
Susan	41	Office manager	High school diploma/GED	Married	2	White	$40,000 to $59,999	Tummy tuck, liposuction	United States
Sylvia	35	Leasing agent	High school diploma/GED	Divorced, remarried	2	Hispanic	$20,000 to $39,999	Breast augmentation, tummy tuck, liposuction, arm lift	Mexico
Taylor	25	College student	Bachelor's degree in progress	Single	0	Hispanic	Less than $19,999	Liposuction	Colombia
Vanessa	27	College student and part-time cosmetologist	Bachelor's degree in progress	Single	1	East Asian	$20,000 to $39,999	Breast augmentation	United States

Note: Demographics were current at the time of interview. Occupation is full time unless otherwise indicated as part time. Annual personal income is self-reported and could include salary and other sources, such as investment income. For unemployed participants, it is based on last salary when previously employed.

Notes

Chapter 1

1. All names of study participants are pseudonyms.

2. Jamaluddin 2015.

3. McGee 2005; Weber 2009.

4. Jones 2008.

5. Weber 2009.

6. Bartky 1988.

7. On black beauty ideals, see Craig 2002, and on lesbian appearance norms, see Faderman 1991.

8. See Bartky 1990; Bordo 2004; and Wolf 1992.

9. See Bartky 1988.

10. Norton et al. 1996.

11. For a thorough overview of the research on the benefits of physical attractiveness and the drawbacks of physical unattractiveness, see Hamermesh 2011; and Rhode 2010.

12. For example, Katherine Mason (2012) finds that for women of size, compared with men of size, income disadvantages persist over time. For a comprehensive review on bias and discrimination against people of size in general, see Puhl and Heuer 2009.

13. Shilling 2012, 4 (emphasis in original).

14. Shilling 2012.

15. Bordo 2004.

16. Unless indicated otherwise, the data in this section come from the American Society of Plastic Surgeons "2017 Plastic Surgery Statistics Report" (ASPS 2018). The ASPS maintains that its data are valid at a 95 percent confidence level with a ±4.05 percent margin of error. For more on the study's methodology and validity, see ASPS 2018, 4.

17. The ASPS describes itself as a nonprofit organization that "supports members in their efforts to provide the highest quality patient care through education, research and advocacy" (ASPS 2018, 3).

18. U.S. Census Bureau 2018.

19. The ASPS uses five age categories—thirteen to nineteen, twenty to twenty-nine, thirty to thirty-nine, forty to fifty-four, and fifty-five and older (ASPS 2018).

20. Prendergast et al. 2011.

21. On the relationship between ethnic and racial minorities and socioeconomic status, see American Psychological Association, n.d.

22. See, e.g., Collins 2000; and Parker et al. 1995.

23. McHugh and Chrisler 2015; Riessman 1983.

24. Conrad 1992, 209.

25. Kaw 1993; Morgan 1991; Sullivan 2001.

26. Markey and Markey 2015.

27. On medicalization, cosmetic surgery, and aging, see Brooks 2017.

28. Edmonds 2011.

29. See Markey and Markey 2015.

30. Markey and Markey 2015, 213.

31. Edmonds 2009, 21.

32. Garcia-Navarro 2014.

33. Davis 1995.

34. Edmonds 2013.

35. Stafford, La Puma, and Schiedermayer 1989.

36. Morgan 1991.

37. Kaw 1993.

38. Dull and West 1991.

39. Brooks 2004; Morgan 1991; Naugler 2010; Tait 2007.

40. Naugler 2010, 119, 120.

41. See Tait 2007, which discusses *Nip/Tuck* (FX) and *Extreme Makeover* (ABC), and Banet-Weiser and Portwood-Stacer 2006, which discusses *Extreme Makeover, I Want a Famous Face* (MTV), and *The Swan* (Fox).

42. Morgan 1991.

43. See Gimlin 2012; Jones 2008; and Sanchez Taylor 2012.

44. Morgan 1991, 41.

45. Erving Goffman (1963) refers to various sources of stigma including abominations of the body, blemishes of character, and tribal status differences.

46. Haiken 1997, 1–2.

47. Adams 2012.

48. See Josh Adams's (2012) discussion on the role of professional organizations in reducing stigma in disreputable industries.

49. See Adams 2012; and Haiken 1997.

50. Adams 2012.

51. Adams 2012; Sullivan 2001.

52. Morgan 1991, 28.

53. Kim, Kim, and Mitra 1997; Tanna et al. 2010.

54. These organizations include the American Society of Plastic Surgeons and the American Society for Aesthetic Plastic Surgery. See Tanne 2003.

55. Denadai et al. 2015.

56. Seattle Plastic Surgery 2013. This surgeon was not part of our study and not a surgeon discussed by our participants.

57. Gilman 1999; Haiken 1997.

58. See Delinsky 2005; and Tam et al. 2012. Kim-Pong Tam and colleagues (2012) document negative attitudes associated with cosmetic surgery across multiple cultures—Hong Kong, Japan, and the United States—and observe that attitudes were less negative in the United States because social contact with someone who has undergone cosmetic surgery is more prevalent in the United States than in these other countries.

59. Motakef et al. 2014, 854e.

60. Stuart, Kurz, and Ashby 2012.

61. Stuart, Kurz, and Ashby 2012, 410.

62. Stuart, Kurz, and Ashby 2012, 411.

63. Stuart, Kurz, and Ashby 2012, 410, 412.

64. Funk, Kennedy, and Sciupac 2016.

65. Anderson 2016. The remaining 84 percent maintain that there is either a neutral benefit or downside (54 percent) or that there are more downsides than benefits (26 percent). The report notes that more favorable views correlate with either having undergone such procedures or having a close family member or friend who has.

66. Anderson 2016. This research is based on a panel of randomly selected adults living in U.S. households and is therefore considered nationally representative.

67. Hunter makes a case that people of color are increasingly willing to undergo cosmetic surgery procedures, reflecting a desire to purchase "racial capital," which she describes as a resource drawn from the body within the context of existing racial hierarchies (2011, 145). Racial capital, Hunter maintains, can be related to skin tone, facial features, and body shape, among other bodily characteristics.

68. See Tait 2007.

69. Brooks 2004, 215–216; Tait 2007, 131.

70. Tait 2007.

71. Braithwaite 2002.

72. Gill 2007b.

73. Anderson 2015. Rosalind Gill (2007b, 152) makes the important observation that this sexual subjectivity exists in a culture in which sexual violence is endemic and only some (namely, young, slim, and beautiful) women are constructed as active, desiring sexual subjects. We make no claims about Kardashian's views on feminism. In fact, at least one journalist has pointed out her controversial relationship to feminism. See Cooper 2018.

74. Hakim 2010; Lehrman 1997.

75. Braun 2009; Gill 2007a.

76. Negra 2009.

77. Whelehan 2010.

78. Nash and Grant 2015.

79. Whelehan 2010, 156. See also Anderson 2015; Gill 2007b; McRobbie 2009; and Negra 2009.

80. Banet-Weiser and Portwood-Stacer 2006, 269.

81. Davis 1995. On the relationship between beauty practices, including cosmetic surgery, and various forms of capital, including racial capital, see Hunter 2002, 2011.

82. Gimlin 2000.

83. Davis 1995.

84. Dull and West 1991; Gillespie 1996. Even Davis (1995), whose interpretation of cosmetic surgery makes central women's agency and choice, acknowledges that choices are bounded.

85. Braun 2009.

86. Braun 2009; Morgan 1991.

87. Bordo 2004; Dull and West 1991; Hunter 2002, 2005, 2011; Kaw 1993; Wolf 1992.

88. Bartky 1988.

89. See Gagné and McGaughey 2002; and Sischo and Yancey Martin 2015.

90. See Weitz 2001.

91. Gagné and McGaughey 2002.

92. Women who could get cosmetic surgery but do not may still symbolically exhibit "embodied resistance," even if they are not necessarily making a conscious choice to oppose hegemonic beauty ideals. See Bobel and Kwan 2011.

93. In other words, cosmetic surgery involves "structurally reproductive agency" rather than "structurally transformative agency." See Hays 1994, 63, 64.

94. Bartky 1988; Wolf 1992.

95. The concept was originally used to account for why proletariats internalize bourgeoisie ideology and are unable to recognize their class oppression and exploitation. See Lukács (1923) 1971. A similar argument can be made that women who have cosmetic surgery are unable to recognize their own oppres-

sion by patriarchal and capitalist forces. For more on cosmetic surgery, false consciousness, and the male gaze, see Gagné and McGaughey 2002.

96. The male gaze involves depicting women as sexual objects for the pleasure of a male viewer; it depicts the world from a masculine heterosexual perspective. See Mulvey 1989.

97. Jeffreys 2015.

98. On racism, see the work of Michael Omi and Howard Winant (1994), whose racial formation theory reformulates the concept, recognizing it as fluid because social structures and discourses themselves are dynamic and subject to rearticulation. For early writings on sexism and women as "other," see Friedan 1963; and de Beauvoir (1949) 2009. The term *ageism* was coined by Robert Butler (1969) to capture prejudice by age group. The disabilities scholar Simi Linton maintains that the terms *ableist* and *ableism* are useful concepts that capture "the centering and domination of the nondisabled experience and point of view" (1998, 8). She extends this understanding of ableism to include the notion that a person's disability determines their abilities or characteristics and that people with disabilities as a collective are inferior to nondisabled people. For an exposition of class politics, particularly as it intersects with race and racial politics, see hooks 2000.

99. Dull and West 1991; Gilman 1999; Hunter 2011; Kaw 1993.

100. Bartky 1988.

101. Pitts-Taylor 2007, 98.

102. Pitts-Taylor 2009, 127.

103. Pitts-Taylor 2009.

104. See American Board of Cosmetic Surgery, n.d. The board refers to the repairing-defects type of surgery as plastic surgery, not cosmetic surgery. While we borrow the board's definition, we recognize the socially constructed nature of the concepts of *defects* and *normal*.

105. Some participants did have these procedures, but not exclusively. A key criterion for study participation was going under the knife.

106. Talley 2014, 5.

107. Social death "describes the cessation of social viability" (Talley 2014, 39). Citing David Sudnow (1967) and Stefan Timmermans (1998), Talley maintains that with social death the patient is treated as a corpse. In this way, social death is intertwined with, and may even expedite, clinical death as, upon designation of social death, treatment of disease or resuscitation efforts often stop.

108. All procedures received Institutional Review Board approval.

109. Participants were compensated fifty dollars for their time.

110. For more on grounded theory, see Charmaz 2014.

111. The first author identifies as an upper-middle-class Asian American. She is thin by cultural standards and has a relatively youthful appearance despite being middle age. She is embedded in athletic and tennis club networks (in both California and Texas) and thus had rapport and credibility with the

upper- and upper-middle-socioeconomic-status participants she interviewed from these circles. The second author is in her early thirties and identifies as white and middle class. She is currently of average size by cultural standards but spent the majority of her life as someone who would be labeled "obese" on the basis of the body mass index. Thus, she was a particularly empathetic listener who was able to establish rapport with her participants.

We both assured participants at the outset of interviews that our role as interviewer was to be a nonjudgmental active listener. At the same time, we acknowledge that our positionality may have limited rapport with some participants. For example, black and Hispanic participants may have been hesitant to discuss race and ethnicity issues with an Asian or white interviewer. However, as a whole, our participants seemed candid, even saying they enjoyed chatting with us about their perspectives and experiences. Moreover, the themes that emerged were consistent across not only both interviewers but women of different backgrounds, suggesting that interviewees' responses were not significantly influenced by interviewer positionality.

112. These percentages sum to 101 percent because of rounding error.

113. These numbers sum to forty-five participants and 98 percent because one retired participant did not report her income.

114. Several of these augmentations were paired with a breast lift.

115. Marianne's face-lift was, she said, a "partial face-lift" that focused mainly on the neck and jowl area.

116. These numbers do not add to forty-six because some women had more than one procedure.

117. Hunter 2002, 2005, 2011.

118. Hunter 2011, 154.

119. The standard deviation is 11.352. Both the mean and the standard deviation are estimates based on self-reported ages. Given the retrospective nature of interviews, it was not uncommon for women to approximate their age at first surgery.

120. These later surgeries sometimes blurred the line between elective and compulsory because some physical problems such as leakage are harmful and require medical intervention.

Chapter 2

1. We do not provide descriptive statistics on the time spent contemplating surgery because many of the women interviewed were not able to provide specifics. Instead, they used descriptors such as "for a while," "years," and a "long time coming."

2. Nationally representative data on deaths related to cosmetic surgery is difficult to come by. However, one study (Bucknor et al. 2018) examining national mortality rates after outpatient cosmetic surgery found that between

2012 and 2017, there were forty-two deaths, the majority of which were from abdominoplasty either in isolation or in combination with breast surgery or facial surgery.

3. American Society for Aesthetic Plastic Surgery 2018.

4. Similarly, we observed large ranges for what they paid for liposuction (about $5,000 to $20,000) and rhinoplasty (about $4,700 to $12,000). We do not provide descriptive statistics on the cost of surgery as participants often provided a range or an approximation, not an exact figure. Also, when participants underwent multiple surgeries simultaneously, they were not aware of the costs of each specific procedure. The approximations reported here do not account for "corrective" procedures, which were at times offered by doctors at a discount.

5. For some, this included using CareCredit, a type of health care credit card available to patients for a range of procedures, from chiropractic services to LASIK. See the CareCredit website, at https://www.carecredit.com/.

6. The exception was Kali. She was paid $600 to have a mini abdominoplasty as part of a clinical trial in California.

7. For a concise summary of both sides, refer to Gagné and McGaughey 2002; and Heyes and Jones 2009.

8. A few of our participants also expressed physical motivations for pursuing surgery. Specifically, they spoke about physical health and physical comfort. For example, Nadine, who had liposuction, said, "It's not healthy to have belly fat." Parvina and Linda, who both had nose surgery to correct a deviated septum and to have their nose sculpted for aesthetic purposes, discussed how surgery enhanced smell and breathing. Casey, who had bilateral breast reduction surgery, said that while she did not currently experience back or shoulder pain, she anticipated it. Sleeping with her boyfriend, she shared, would also cause physical discomfort as he would, at times, roll over and pin down her breast. Finally, Chloe, who had a thigh tuck, said her thighs had been physically uncomfortable, and she would get rashes from chafing.

9. See, e.g., Davis 1991; Gimlin 2000; Saxena 2013; and Sischo and Yancey Martin 2015.

10. *Normative femininity* is defined as the norms and social expectations regarding female appearance and behavior that women are held to. See Bartky 1988. A good example of a beauty practice that produces normative femininity is women's body hair removal. See Fahs 2011; and Toerien, Wilkinson, and Choi 2005.

11. See, e.g., Davis 1995; Saxena 2013; and Sischo and Yancey Martin 2015.

12. West and Zimmerman 1987, 136.

13. See Bartky 1988.

14. Peter Paul Rubens is a Flemish artist who is known for painting larger women (or women who by today's standard might be described as "plus-size").

The term "Rubenesque" is still used today to capture full-figured women. For a brief history of feminine beauty ideals, see Howard and Ginsburg 2018.

15. Robehmed 2018. According to the Hollywood source *Heightline*, Jenner is 5'10", weighs 119 pounds, and has bust and waist measurements of 34 inches and 24 inches, respectively. See "Kendall Jenner" 2015.

16. We discuss bra-size increases instead of implant size in cubic centimeters because the majority of participants who had breast surgery discussed their breast size increase using the former, not the latter.

17. Young 1992.

18. At the same time, there are limits to what are considered sexy breasts, illustrating the narrowness of cultural circumscriptions of femininity. Casey's reasons for surgery show her awareness of these narrow definitions of beauty. At age forty, she underwent liposuction and had both breasts reduced to the equivalent of a 34D bra. Referring to her original 34DDD breasts as "freak town," she lamented the cultural double standard associated with women's breasts. She said, "I think I look pretty good for forty and a little bit still sexy if I still choose to. I didn't want to be that fifty-year-old woman with big boobs because then you kind of get frumpy and, as I said, matronly really quickly." She continued, "You go from sex bot to matronly almost overnight." Thus, while breasts are a defining feature of womanhood, if they are too large, sagging, or formless, they are recoded as matronly and unattractive.

19. For an evolutionary psychology perspective, see Etcoff 2000.

20. See Bordo 2004; and Wolf 1992.

21. The sociologist Harold Garfinkel coined the term to describe compliance with dominant cultural norms and scripts. According to Garfinkel, a cultural dope is a person "who produces the stable features of the society by acting in compliance with preestablished and legitimate alternatives of action that the common culture provides" (1967, 68).

22. See, e.g., Saxena 2013.

23. See Puhl and Heuer 2009.

24. Kwan 2010.

25. On the generalized other, see Mead 1934.

26. For an overview, see Rhode 2010.

27. See Gimlin 2013; and Jones 2008.

28. Ladd is an American actress who played an "angel" in the hit ABC series *Charlie's Angels*. The series ran from 1976 to 1981.

29. Johns Hopkins Medicine, n.d.

30. American Academy of Cosmetic Surgery, n.d.

31. Parsons 1951.

32. Crandall 1994.

33. See Bartky 1988.

34. See Bartky 1988; Dellinger and Williams 1997; Fahs 2011; and Wolf 1992.

35. On the social sanctions associated with breaking embodiment norms, see Bobel and Kwan 2011, 2019.

36. Centers for Disease Control and Prevention 2019.

37. National Organization for Women, n.d.

38. See Craig 2002.

39. Stanley 2017.

40. See the website of the Dove Self-Esteem Project, at https://www.dove.com/us/en/dove-self-esteem-project.html.

41. See Hanbury 2018.

42. See Crehan 2016.

Chapter 3

1. The surgery was a combination of septoplasty and rhinoplasty. Her surgery was mostly covered by health insurance, although Jenna informed us that there were billing problems because of mismanaged paperwork, and for some time, she was concerned that she would owe about $15,000 for the procedure.

2. We revisit this in Chapter 4 in our discussion of how participants distance themselves from surgeries of which they disapprove.

3. *Botched* is an American reality television series that premiered on E! in the summer of 2014. It follows two cosmetic surgeons as they attempt to correct cosmetic surgery procedures that have gone wrong—were botched.

4. American Society of Plastic Surgeons (ASPS, n.d.) lists the types of breast implants available to patients as saline, structured saline, silicone, gummy bear, round, smooth, and textured.

5. See WebMD 2019a.

6. WebMD maintains that silicone gel and saline implants do not have significant differences in safety but points out that each type of breast implant has its pros and cons. The Food and Drug Administration, however, allows women only ages twenty-two and older to obtain silicone gel breast implants, "citing the issues surrounding the removal of ruptured silicone gel breast implants." WebMD 2019b.

7. *Dictionary.com*, s.v. "natural," available at https://www.dictionary.com/browse/natural?s=t.

8. "'The Talk' Ladies" 2012.

9. Like participants' names, doctors' names are also pseudonyms.

10. Kali, who had abdominoplasty, had a similar but slightly different perspective to Lacy's that is noteworthy. While Lacy discussed sculpting the body naturally through diet and exercise, Kali's understanding of *natural* includes surgery. This is because she feels the results of her cosmetic surgery are similar to something that she could have done without surgery. In her words, "That's still something you could've done on your own." She further remarked that even if one's body hits a plateau with weight loss, one can continue to lose weight. "Plateaus aren't forever. Something could've changed that; might as well have

been surgery. Someone could take a supplement, or change their diet, or change their exercise plan." For this reason, Kali thinks of her body as natural because she believes her weight loss could have been achieved without surgery. All she did was find a way off the plateau she had hit. In her case, it was surgery that allowed her body to continue its natural (weight-loss) trajectory.

11. Berkowitz 2017, 157 (emphasis in original).

12. Gimlin 2013; Jones 2008; Sanchez Taylor 2012.

13. Gummy bear implants are a type of form-stable implants that maintain their shape even when the implant shell is broken (ASPS, n.d.).

14. Dicker 2013.

15. Because of our grounded theory approach, we asked only thirty-five participants if they viewed their postoperative *bodies* as natural. About 70 percent of these participants said they do, while about 30 percent said they do not.

16. Lavanna's perspective corresponds with an empirical reality that breast implants require checkups, as well as even a possible replacement. The American Society of Plastic Surgeons acknowledges a 2011 report by the Food and Drug Administration on the safety of silicone implants that documents that one in five patients needed a replacement or revision on their breast implants after ten years. However, the American Society of Plastic Surgeons stresses that this means four in five did not and that these later procedures are not always because of deflation or rupture, stating that "many revisions are by choice, when women decide they want to change their size or have further refinement" (Lawton 2018).

17. See Goffman 1963.

18. Goffman 1959, 1963.

19. See Gimlin 2000; Saxena 2013; and Sischo and Yancey Martin 2015.

20. Gilman 1999; Saxena 2013.

Chapter 4

1. The term *boundary work* is attributed to Thomas Gieryn (1983, 1999), a sociologist who discussed the demarcation of science from nonscience. In Gieryn's analysis, boundary work enables science to distinguish itself from less authoritative nonscience, thereby establishing epistemic authority and professional autonomy. Scholars have extended the concept to include moral boundaries and identity work (e.g., Lamont 1992). For an overview of boundary work, see Lamont and Molnár 2002.

2. See, e.g., Gimlin 2010, 2012; and Saxena 2013.

3. Talley 2014.

4. On cultural discourses about fat and obesity, see Kwan and Graves 2013.

5. We acknowledge that a few participants wished they had done more research on their doctors. Several felt that the consulting fee (typically $100 or higher) limited the extent they could vet doctors. The majority of participants, however, were generally pleased with their choice of doctor.

6. Parvina admitted to having one reservation about undergoing surgery abroad. If something should go wrong with surgery, she felt she would likely not be able to sue the surgeon. "My sister had her nose done here. He's the best Beverly Hills Persian plastic surgeon. He did the queen of Iran back in the nineties. . . . My fear was, if someone messes up your nose here, you can sue them and go after their license. You're kind of screwed when you're going abroad. You have to really trust them."

7. While scholars typically think of status characteristics in terms of race, ethnicity, gender, sex, sexuality, age, ability, and class, Murray Webster and James Driskell (1983) write that beauty operates in a similar manner to other status characteristics.

8. Silva et al. 2016.

9. Huis in 't Veld, Canales, and Furnas 2017.

10. Kang 2010.

11. Petersen 1966.

12. An analysis by Meera Deo and colleagues (2008) of prime-time TV programs on national broadcast networks found overwhelming depictions of Asian and Pacific Islander Americans as, among other stereotypes, ideal workers, scholastic overachievers, and geeky science and computer nerds. These researchers also found that more than half the characters in their sample held high-status occupations, many of which required advanced degrees such as an MD.

13. Some research has found high rates of mental disorders among people seeking cosmetic surgery. Jun Ishigooka and colleagues (1998) found that nearly 50 percent of their sample (of 415) exhibited clinically diagnosable mental disorders and about 55 percent exhibited poor social adjustment. Randy Sansone and Lori Sansone (2007) document a heightened risk of suicide among women following breast augmentation surgery, along with a high prevalence of body dysmorphic disorder and associated comorbidities.

14. Rebecca was not able to specify how many operations she had, even when pressed, merely saying it was "many."

15. Gimlin 2010.

16. Verner 2011.

17. See Braun 2009 on cosmetic surgery, choice, and empowerment.

18. Throsby 2008.

19. See King et al. 2017.

20. See Snow and Anderson 1987, 1348.

21. Young 1992.

Chapter 5

1. Honigman, Phillips, and Castle 2004; Sarwer et al. 2005.

2. For examples of these, see the TV shows *Botched* (surgeries gone wrong) and *Extreme Makeover* and *The Swan* (wildly successful surgeries).

3. Although we talked to all participants about their postoperative sentiments, we do not give the percentage of our sample who were content with
surgery. Our sample is based on nonprobability sampling strategies, and we do
not want to intimate that such levels of contentment would be found in a larger
population of women who have undergone invasive cosmetic surgery. Moreover,
contentment with surgery is not an all-or-nothing phenomenon. As we illustrate,
even though the majority of our participants had a positive attitude and experience with surgery, they also expressed disappointments across the life course.

4. On the male gaze, see Mulvey 1989.

5. See the work of Naomi Wolf (1992), who argues that these beauty ideologies correspond to women's political achievement, and these ideologies function as a means of holding women back—a form of oppression to counter their
political advancements.

6. See Bonafini and Pozzilli 2010 on shifting ideals of female beauty.

7. U.S. Food and Drug Administration 2019.

8. The study examined only silicone gel breast implants. See U.S. Food and
Drug Administration 2011.

9. Mayo Clinic 2017.

10. A MRSA infection results from "a type of staph bacteria that's become
resistant to many of the antibiotics used to treat ordinary staph infections."
Mayo Clinic 2018.

11. U.S. Food and Drug Administration 2019.

12. U.S. Food and Drug Administration 2018.

13. WebMD 2019c.

14. American Board of Cosmetic Surgery 2016.

15. See American Psychological Association, n.d.

16. L'Oréal, n.d.

17. Anthony 2018.

18. Festinger 1957.

19. We acknowledge the influence of self-selection. It is possible that women
who have positive experiences with cosmetic surgery are more likely to volun-
teer to participate in a study like ours.

20. Interestingly, the doctor who performed the rhinoplasty in 1987 billed the
procedure as a deviated septum. When asked if she had problems breathing, she
said definitively, "Oh no, but that was back in the days the doctors could do that."

21. The first author conducted this interview.

22. Bartky 1988; Jeffreys 2015; Wolf 1992.

Chapter 6

1. Chu and Posner 2013; Geiger and Parker 2018; Pew Research Center 2018.

2. Chu and Posner 2013; Geiger and Parker 2018; Pew Research Center 2018;
Smith et al. 2018.

3. Wolf 1992.

4. Ferreiro, Seoane, and Senra 2011; Paxton et al. 2006; Runfola et al. 2013.

5. Bartky 1988; Jeffreys 2015; Wolf 1992.

6. Bartky 1988; Bordo 2004; Jeffreys 2015; Wolf 1992.

7. Jones 2008.

8. Davis 1991, 1995.

9. See Gill 2007a, 2007b.

10. See Kwan and Trautner 2009; Rhode 2010; and Webster and Driskell 1983.

11. Following Pitts-Taylor 2007.

12. On cultural normalization, see Brooks 2004; Morgan 1991; Naugler 2010; and Tait 2007. On the medicalization of women's body image, see Markey and Markey 2015.

13. West and Zimmerman 1987.

14. Sandra Bartky (1988) maintains that women's beauty ideals are homogenizing despite rhetoric to the contrary. Brenda Weber (2009) argues specifically that cosmetic surgery has a homogenizing effect.

15. See, e.g., Rodin, Silberstein, and Striegel-Moore 1984.

16. See, e.g., Davis 1995.

17. Haiken 1997.

18. See Gimlin 2013; Jones 2008; and Sanchez Taylor 2012.

19. See, e.g., Brooks 2004; Morgan 1991; Naugler 2010; and Tait 2007.

20. For example, with the medicalization of body weight, doctors now use metrics such as the body mass index or waist circumference to place patients in diagnostic categories such as clinically overweight or obese. Those thusly labeled are then provided medically sanctioned steps to address their condition (e.g., change their diet and physical activity levels, take weight-loss drugs, obtain bariatric surgery). See Blackburn 2011.

21. Kvaale, Haslam, and Gottdiener 2013.

22. The grand question is whether body image can be "fixed" using medicine. See Markey and Markey 2015.

23. ASPS 2018.

24. Anderson 2016.

25. Kim, Kim, and Mitra 1997; Tanna et al. 2010.

26. Stuart, Kurz, and Ashby 2012.

27. See, e.g., Saxena 2013.

28. See Collins 2000; and Parker et al. 1995.

29. See, e.g., Molloy and Herzberger 1998.

30. Swami, Nogueira Campana, and Coles 2012. Specifically, these researchers compared Caucasians, South Asians, and African Caribbeans. They acknowledge, however, that ethnicity accounts for only a small proportion of the variance in attitudes, and that body appreciation and self-esteem are stronger predictors.

31. Goffman 1963.

32. On stigma management and gay or bisexual men with HIV/AIDS, see Siegel, Lune, and Meyer 1998. On stigma management and voluntary childlessness, see Park 2002.

33. Including neutralizations, accounts, and passing. See Goffman 1963; Scott and Lyman 1968; and Sykes and Matza 1957.

34. Deviance exemplars "demarcate identity by setting up a 'straw man' or a 'straw woman' to whom one can compare herself" (Ronai 1994, 203). They are concepts people use to compare themselves to others. For example, some overweight women categorically reject negative labels associated with the overweight category—for example, that they are physically unattractive—and resist the trait the exemplar represents. See Cordell and Ronai 1999.

35. See, e.g., Kwan 2010. Passing involves the "management of undisclosed discrediting information about self" (Goffman 1963, 42).

36. DeJong 1980.

37. Gimlin 2000, 81.

38. Gimlin 2000, 81.

39. Saxena 2013, 365.

40. Gimlin 2007. On narrative accounts, also see Scott and Lyman 1968.

41. Gimlin 2007.

42. Saxena 2013.

43. Sischo and Yancey Martin 2015. Josh Adams (2010) also examines motivational narratives and accounts of cosmetic surgery.

44. Dull and West 1991.

45. For more on this term, see Pitts-Taylor 2007.

46. On the surgical other, see Gimlin 2010, 2012.

47. Gimlin 2012, 108.

48. See Gimlin 2010, 2012. Debra Gimlin's cross-cultural findings are particularly important because she observes that women's use of accounts is shaped by cultural repertoires that are geographically informed. For example, American women are more likely to use socioeconomic boundaries to determine the appropriateness of surgery compared with women in Great Britain.

49. Saxena 2013, 355.

50. See, e.g., Gimlin 2000, 2013; Sanchez Taylor 2012; Saxena 2013; and Sischo and Yancey Martin 2015.

51. Davis 1995; Gimlin 2013; Pitts-Taylor 2007.

52. See, e.g., Carruthers et al. 2007; and Hoffman 2015.

53. See Kates and Shaw-Garlock 1999; and Thompson and Haytko 1997.

54. Bartky (1988) illustrates this point at length, showing the many extensive and elaborate body management processes with which women engage.

55. Weisman, 2012.

56. Thompson and Haytko 1997, 33.

57. See Gimlin 2000; Saxena 2013; and Sischo and Yancey Martin 2015.

58. Gilman 1999; Kaw 1993; Saxena 2013.

59. Sanchez Taylor 2012.

60. Gimlin 2013, 922.

61. Conspicuous consumption is a concept first developed by Thorstein Veblen ([1899] 1994) to capture the notion that people spend money on luxury goods and services to display their wealth and income.

62. Gimlin 2013, 930.

63. Gimlin 2013; Sanchez Taylor 2012.

64. U.S. Department of Health and Human Services 2017.

65. Gieryn 1983.

66. Epstein 1992, 232.

67. Lamont, Pendergrass, and Pachucki 2015, 853.

68. Talley 2014.

69. Rhode 2010.

70. See, e.g., Bacon and Aphramor 2011.

71. See Puhl and Heuer 2009.

72. Mann et al. 2007.

73. Ray 2018.

74. Ray 2018, 469.

75. See, e.g., Shannon 2018; "Dr Bumbum" 2018.

76. Petersen 1966.

77. Kang 2010.

78. Throsby 2008.

79. Gimlin 2010.

80. Gimlin 2010, 67–68. Gimlin argues that surgeons too construct narratives of the self in these social processes.

81. The one exception to this was Michael Jackson, whom about an equal number of women of color and white participants invoked as an example of "bad" cosmetic surgery.

82. de Beauvoir (1949) 2009. For example, in the case of gender, *woman* is defined in reference to the normative *man* and is categorically distinct from man.

83. The latter is somewhat racially ambiguous. However, she is married to, and has children with, the African American rapper Kanye West. We acknowledge that Kim Kardashian has been accused of cultural appropriation for styling her hair in cornrows (Bennett 2018).

84. Akinro and Mbunyuza-Memani 2019; Awad et al. 2015; Baker-Sperry and Grauerholz 2003; Bryant 2013; Jha 2016.

85. Li 2016.

86. See Snow and Anderson 1987, 1348.

87. Talley 2014, 13.

88. Talley 2014, 14.

89. Bartky 1988; Weber 2009.

90. Young 1992.

91. Rape culture is "a complex of beliefs that encourages male sexual aggression and supports violence against women. . . . In a rape culture both men and women assume that sexual violence is a fact of life, inevitable as death or taxes" (Buchwald, Fletcher, and Roth 1993, v). On constitutional and feminist critiques of rape shield laws, see Roman 2011; also see Janzen 2015.

92. On blaming sexual assault victims, see Gravelin, Biernat, and Baldwin 2017; and Gravelin, Biernat, and Bucher 2018.

93. The American Association of University Women reports that slut shaming is one of the most common forms of sexual harassment middle and high school students face. A third of students surveyed reported experiencing unwelcome comments, jokes, or gestures (Hill and Kearl 2011). On slut shaming in cyberspace, see Tanenbaum 2015.

94. Smith et al. 2018.

95. Ashcraft and Stump 2019.

96. Dockterman 2014.

97. Minsberg 2018.

98. Alesali and Zdanowicz 2019.

99. We recognize that some scholars argue that sexual behaviors, including men's aggression and women's passivity, can be framed along evolutionary lines (e.g., Buss and Schmitt 1993). However, we focus instead on what we consider a persuasive interpretive framework—social scripts theory.

100. Simon and Gagnon 1986.

101. Frith 2009.

102. Kim et al. 2007, 146. Their research shows the high rate of these scripts in popular television shows.

103. Frith and Kitzinger 2001.

104. Bareket et al. 2018.

105. Wolf 1997; Young 1993.

106. See Honigman, Phillips, and Castle 2004; and Sarwer et al. 2005.

107. Mull 2019.

108. Paquette and Raine 2004.

109. See, e.g., Kaiser, Freeman, and Wingate 1985; and Kwan 2010.

110. Baker-Sperry and Grauerholz 2003; Baumann 2008; Vannini and Mc-Cright 2004.

111. Anderson et al. 2018; Turner 2011.

112. Leeds 1994.

113. See Leeds 1994, 154–155.

114. Rose Weitz (2001) discusses how accommodation and resistance are inseparable and often come together.

115. Bombak, Monaghan, and Rich 2019.

116. See Mann et al. 2007.

References

Adams, Josh. 2010. "Motivational Narratives and Assessments of the Body after Cosmetic Surgery." *Qualitative Health Research* 20 (6): 755–767.

———. 2012. "Cleaning Up the Dirty Work: Professionalization and the Management of Stigma in the Cosmetic Surgery and Tattoo Industries." *Deviant Behavior* 33 (3): 149–167.

Akinro, Ngozi, and Lindani Mbunyuza-Memani. 2019. "Black Is Not Beautiful: Persistent Messages and the Globalization of 'White' Beauty in African Women's Magazines." *Journal of International and Intercultural Communication* 12 (4): 308–324.

Alesali, Loumay, and Christina Zdanowicz. 2019. "She Told Them Leggings Were Too Suggestive, So They Wore Them in Protest." *CNN*, March 31. Available at https://www.cnn.com/2019/03/28/us/mothers-problem-with-leggings-trnd/index.html.

American Academy of Cosmetic Surgery. n.d. "About Us." Available at https://www.cosmeticsurgery.org/page/About (accessed December 11, 2019).

American Board of Cosmetic Surgery. 2016. "Top 3 Tips for Maintaining Your Cosmetic Surgery Results." May 24. Available at https://www.americanboardcosmeticsurgery.org/top-3-tips-for-maintaining-your-cosmetic-surgery-results/.

———. n.d. "Cosmetic Surgery vs. Plastic Surgery." Available at https://www.americanboardcosmeticsurgery.org/patient-resources/cosmetic-surgery-vs-plastic-surgery/ (accessed December 11, 2019).

American Psychological Association. n.d. "Ethnic and Racial Minorities and Socioeconomic Status." Available at https://www.apa.org/pi/ses/resources/publications/factsheet-erm.pdf (accessed December 11, 2019).

American Society for Aesthetic Plastic Surgery. 2018. "Cosmetic Surgery National Data Bank Statistics, 2017." Available at https://www.surgery.org/sites/default/files/ASAPS-Stats2017.pdf.

Anderson, Joel R., Elise Holland, Courtney Heldreth, and Scott P. Johnson. 2018. "Revisiting the Jezebel Stereotype: The Impact of Target Race on Sexual Objectification." *Psychology of Women Quarterly* 42 (4): 461–476.

Anderson, Kristin J. 2015. *Modern Misogyny: Anti-feminism in a Post-feminist Era*. New York: Oxford University Press.

Anderson, Monica. 2016. "Americans Aren't Sold on Plastic Surgery: Few Have Had It Done, Opinions Mostly Mixed." Pew Research Center, October 18. Available at http://www.pewresearch.org/fact-tank/2016/10/18/americans-arent-sold-on-plastic-surgery-few-have-had-it-done-opinions-mostly-mixed/.

Anthony, Kiara. 2018. "Panniculectomy." *Healthline*, February 26. Available at https://www.healthline.com/health/panniculectomy.

Ashcraft, Lindsey, and Scott Stump. 2019. "Teen Girls at Maryland High School Fight Back after Finding List Ranking Their Looks." *Today*, March 28. Available at https://www.today.com/news/teen-girls-maryland-high-school-fight-back-after-finding-list-t151125.

ASPS (American Society of Plastic Surgeons). 2018. "2017 Plastic Surgery Statistics Report." Available at https://www.plasticsurgery.org/documents/News/Statistics/2017/plastic-surgery-statistics-full-report-2017.pdf.

———. n.d. "Breast Augmentation: Augmentation Mammaplasty." https://www.plasticsurgery.org/cosmetic-procedures/breast-augmentation/implants.

Awad, Germine H., Carolette Norwood, Desire S. Taylor, Mercedes Martinez, Shannon McClain, Bianca Jones, Andrea Holman, and Collette Chapman-Hilliard. 2015. "Beauty and Body Image Concerns among African American College Women." *Journal of Black Psychology* 41 (6): 540–564.

Bacon, Linda, and Lucy Aphramor. 2011. "Weight Science: Evaluating the Evidence for a Paradigm Shift." *Nutrition Journal* 10 (9): 1–13.

Baker-Sperry, Lori, and Liz Grauerholz. 2003. "The Pervasiveness and Persistence of the Feminine Beauty Ideal in Children's Fairy Tales." *Gender and Society* 15 (5): 711–726.

Banet-Weiser, Sarah, and Laura Portwood-Stacer. 2006. "'I Just Want to Be Me Again!' Beauty Pageants, Reality Television and Post-feminism." *Feminist Theory* 7 (2): 255–272.

Bareket, Orly, Rotem Kahalon, Nurit Schnabel, and Peter Glick. 2018. "The Madonna-Whore Dichotomy: Men Who Perceive Women's Nurturance and Sexuality as Mutually Exclusive Endorse Patriarchy and Show Lower Relationship Satisfaction." *Sex Roles* 79 (9–10): 519–532.

Bartky, Sandra Lee. 1988. "Foucault, Femininity, and the Modernization of Pa-triarchal Power." In *Feminism and Foucault: Reflections of Resistance*, edited by Irene Diamond and Lee Quinby, 61–86. Boston: Northeastern University Press.

———. 1990. *Femininity and Domination: Studies in the Phenomenology of Oppression*. New York: Routledge.

Baumann, Shyon. 2008. "The Moral Underpinnings of Beauty: A Meaning-Based Explanation for Light and Dark Complexions in Advertising." *Poetics* 36 (1): 2–23.

Bennett, Jessica. 2018. "Kim Kardashian-West Accused of Cultural Appropriation for Rocking Cornrows." *Ebony*, June 18. Available at https://www.ebony.com/entertainment/kim-kardashian-west-accused-of-cultural-appropriation-for-rocking-cornrows/.

Berkowitz, Dana. 2017. *Botox Nation: Changing the Face of America*. New York: New York University Press.

Blackburn, George L. 2011. "Medicalizing Obesity: Individual, Economic, and Medical Consequences." *AMA Journal of Ethics*, December. Available at https://journalofethics.ama-assn.org/article/medicalizing-obesity-individual-economic-and-medical-consequences/2011-12.

Bobel, Chris, and Samantha Kwan, eds. 2011. *Embodied Resistance: Challenging the Norms, Breaking the Rules*. Nashville, TN: Vanderbilt University Press.

———, eds. 2019. *Body Battlegrounds: Transgressions, Tensions, and Transformations*. Nashville, TN: Vanderbilt University Press.

Bombak, Andrea, Lee F. Monaghan, and Emma Rich. 2019. "Dietary Approaches to Weight-Loss, Health at Every Size® and Beyond: Rethinking the War on Obesity." *Social Theory and Health* 17 (1): 89–108.

Bonafini, B. A., and P. Pozzilli. 2010. "Body Weight and Beauty: The Changing Face of the Ideal Female Body Weight." *Obesity Reviews* 12 (1): 62–65.

Bordo, Susan. 2004. *Unbearable Weight: Feminism, Western Culture, and the Body*. 10th Anniversary ed. Berkeley: University of California Press.

Braithwaite, Ann. 2002. "The Personal, the Political, Third-Wave and Postfeminisms." *Feminist Theory* 3 (3): 335–344.

Braun, Virginia. 2009. "'The Women Are Doing It for Themselves': The Rhetoric of Choice and Agency around Female Genital 'Cosmetic Surgery.'" *Australian Feminist Studies* 24 (60): 233–249.

Brooks, Abigail T. 2004. "'Under the Knife and Proud of It': An Analysis of the Normalization of Cosmetic Surgery." *Critical Sociology* 30 (2): 207–239.

———. 2017. *The Ways Women Age: Using and Refusing Cosmetic Intervention*. New York: New York University Press.

Bryant, Susan L. 2013. "The Beauty Ideal: The Effects of European Standards of Beauty on Black Women." *Columbia Social Work Review* 4:80–91.

Buchwald, Emilie, Pamela R. Fletcher, and Martha Roth, eds. 1993. *Transforming a Rape Culture*. Minneapolis, MN: Milkweed Editions.

Bucknor, Alexandra, Sabine A. Egeler, Austin D. Chen, Anmol Chattha, Parisa Kamali, Gary Brownstein, Lawrence Reed, David Watts, and Samuel J. Lin. 2018. "National Mortality Rates after Outpatient Cosmetic Surgery and Low Rates of Perioperative Deep Vein Thrombosis Screening and Prophylaxis." *Plastic and Reconstructive Surgery* 142 (1): 90–98.

Buss, David M., and David P. Schmitt. 1993. "Sexual Strategies Theory: An Evolutionary Perspective on Human Mating." *Psychological Review* 100 (2): 204–232.

Butler, Robert N. 1969. "Age-ism: Another Form of Bigotry." *The Gerontologist* 9 (4): 243–246.

Carruthers, Alastair, Joel L. Cohen, Sue Ellen Cox, Koenraad De Boulle, Steven Fagien, Charles J. Finn, Timothy Flynn, Nicholas J. Lowe, Hervé Raspaldo, Boris Sommer, and Ada Trindade de Almeida. 2007. "Facial Aesthetics: Achieving the Natural, Relaxed Look." *Journal of Cosmetic and Laser Therapy* 9 (suppl. 1): 6–10.

Centers for Disease Control and Prevention. 2019. "Adult Obesity Causes and Consequences." November 6. Available at https://www.cdc.gov/obesity/adult/causes.html.

Charmaz, Kathy. 2014. *Constructing Grounded Theory*. 2nd ed. Los Angeles: SAGE.

Chu, Anna, and Charles Posner. 2013. "The State of Women in America: A 50-State Analysis of How Women Are Faring across the Nation." Center for American Progress, September 25. Available at https://www.americanprogress.org/issues/women/reports/2013/09/25/74836/the-state-of-women-in-america/.

Collins, Patricia Hill. 2000. *Black Feminist Thought: Knowledge, Consciousness, and the Politics of Empowerment*. Rev. 2nd ed. New York: Routledge.

Conrad, Peter. 1992. "Medicalization and Social Control." *Annual Review of Sociology* 18:209–232.

Cooper, Kelly-Leigh. 2018. "Kim Kardashian: Feminist Icon or Emoji Opportunist?" *BBC News*, March 8. Available at https://www.bbc.com/news/world-us-canada-43330016.

Cordell, Gina, and Carol Rambo Ronai. 1999. "Identity Management among Overweight Women: Narrative Resistance to Stigma." In *Interpreting Weight: The Social Management of Fatness and Thinness*, edited by Jeffery Sobal and Donna Maurer, 29–47. New York: Aldine de Gruyter.

Craig, Maxine Leeds. 2002. *Ain't I a Beauty Queen? Black Women, Beauty, and the Politics of Race*. New York: Oxford University Press.

Crandall, Christian. 1994. "Prejudice against Fat People: Ideology and Self-Interest." *Journal of Personality and Social Psychology* 66 (5): 882–894.

Crehan, Maddy. 2016. "Embrace the Body Image Movement." Victorian Women's Trust, July 28. Available at https://www.vwt.org.au/embrace-the-body-image-movement/.

Davis, Kathy. 1991. "Remaking the She-Devil: A Critical Look at Feminist Approaches to Beauty." *Hypatia* 6 (2): 21–43.

———. 1995. *Reshaping the Female Body: The Dilemma of Cosmetic Surgery.* New York: Routledge.

de Beauvoir, Simone. (1949) 2009. *The Second Sex.* Translated by Constance Borde and Sheila Malovany-Chevallier. New York: Vintage Books.

DeJong, William. 1980. "The Stigma of Obesity: The Consequences of Naïve Assumptions Concerning the Causes of Physical Deviance." *Journal of Health and Social Behavior* 21 (1): 75–87.

Delinsky, Sherrie Selwyn. 2005. "Cosmetic Surgery: A Common and Accepted Form of Self-Improvement?" *Journal of Applied Social Psychology* 35 (10): 2012–2028.

Dellinger, Kirsten, and Christine L. Williams. 1997. "Makeup at Work: Negotiating Appearance Rules in the Workplace." *Gender and Society* 11 (2): 151–177.

Denadai, Rafael, Karin Milleni Araujo, Hugo Samartine Junior, Rodrigo Denadai, and Cassio Eduardo Raposo-Amaral. 2015. "Aesthetic Surgery Reality Television Shows: Do They Influence Public Perception of the Scope of Plastic Surgery?" *Aesthetic Plastic Surgery* 39 (6): 1000–1009.

Deo, Meera E., Jenny J. Lee, Christina B. Chin, Noriko Milman, and Nancy Wang Yuen. 2008. "Missing in Action: 'Framing' Race on Prime-Time Television." *Social Justice* 35 (2): 145–162.

Dicker, Ron. 2013. "American Bra Size Average Increases from 34B to 34DD in Just 20 Years, Survey Says." *Huffington Post,* July 24. Available at https://www.huffingtonpost.com/2013/07/24/bra-size-survey_n_3645267.html.

Dockterman, Eliana. 2014. "How 'Hot or Not' Created the Internet We Know Today." *Time,* June 18. Available at http://time.com/2894727/hot-or-not-internet/.

"Dr Bumbum, Brazil Cosmetic Surgeon, Charged with Murder." 2018. *BBC News,* August 16. Available at https://www.bbc.com/news/world-latin-america-45203740.

Dull, Diana, and Candace West. 1991. "Accounting for Cosmetic Surgery: The Accomplishment of Gender." *Social Problems* 38 (1): 54–70.

Edmonds, Alexander. 2009. "Beauty, Health and Risk in Brazilian Plastic Surgery." *Medische Antropologie* 21 (1): 21–38.

———. 2011. "Surgery as Therapy." *New York Times,* August 14. Available at https://archive.nytimes.com/query.nytimes.com/gst/fullpage-9F0CE2D61739F937A2575BC0A9679D8B63.html.

———. 2013. "Can Medicine Be Aesthetic?" *Medical Anthropology Quarterly* 27 (2): 233–252.

Epstein, Cynthia Fuchs. 1992. "Tinker-Bells and Pinups: The Construction and Reconstruction of Gender Boundaries at Work." In *Cultivating Differences: Symbolic Boundaries and the Making of Inequality,* edited by Michèle

Lamont and Marcel Fournier, 232–256. Chicago: University of Chicago Press.

Etcoff, Nancy. 2000. *Survival of the Prettiest: The Science of Beauty.* New York: Anchor.

Faderman, Lillian. 1991. *Odd Girls and Twilight Lovers: A History of Lesbian Life in Twentieth-Century America.* New York: Columbia University Press.

Fahs, Breanne. 2011. "Dreaded 'Otherness': Heteronormative Patrolling in Women's Body Hair Rebellions." *Gender and Society* 25 (4): 451–472.

Ferreiro, Fátima, Gloria Seoane, and Carmen Senra. 2011. "A Prospective Study of Risk Factors for the Development of Depression and Disordered Eating in Adolescents." *Journal of Clinical Child and Adolescent Psychology* 40 (3): 500–505.

Festinger, Leon. 1957. *A Theory of Cognitive Dissonance.* Stanford, CA: Stanford University Press.

Friedan, Betty. 1963. *The Feminine Mystique.* New York: W. W. Norton.

Frith, Hannah. 2009. "Sexual Scripts, Sexual Refusals, and Rape." In *Rape: Challenging Contemporary Thinking,* edited by Miranda Horvath and Jennifer Brown, 99–122. Devon, UK: Willan.

Frith, Hannah, and Celia Kitzinger. 2001. "Reformulating Sexual Script Theory: Developing a Discursive Psychology of Sexual Negotiation." *Theory and Psychology* 11 (2): 209–232.

Funk, Cary, Brian Kennedy, and Elizabeth Podrebarac Sciupac. 2016. "U.S. Public Wary of Biomedical Technologies to 'Enhance' Human Abilities." Pew Research Center, July 26. Available at https://www.pewresearch.org/science/2016/07/26/u-s-public-wary-of-biomedical-technologies-to-enhance-human-abilities/.

Gagné, Patricia, and Deanna McGaughey. 2002. "Designing Women: Cultural Hegemony and the Exercise of Power among Women Who Have Undergone Elective Mammoplasty." *Gender and Society* 16 (6): 814–838.

Garcia-Navarro, Lulu. 2014. "In Brazil, Nips and Tucks Don't Raise an Eyebrow." *NPR,* October 7. Available at https://www.npr.org/sections/parallels/2014/10/07/353270270/an-uplifting-story-brazils-obsession-with-plastic-surgery.

Garfinkel, Harold. 1967. *Studies in Ethnomethodology.* Englewood Cliffs, NJ: Prentice Hall.

Geiger, A. W., and Kim Parker. 2018. "For Women's History Month, a Look at Gender Gains—and Gaps—in the U.S." Pew Research Center, March 15. Available at http://www.pewresearch.org/fact-tank/2018/03/15/for-womens-history-month-a-look-at-gender-gains-and-gaps-in-the-u-s/.

Gieryn, Thomas F. 1983. "Boundary-Work and the Demarcation of Science from Non-science: Strains and Interests in Professional Interests of Scientists." *American Sociological Review* 48:781–795.

———. 1999. *Cultural Boundaries of Science: Credibility on the Line.* Chicago: University of Chicago Press.

Gill, Rosalind. 2007a. "Critical Respect: The Difficulties and Dilemmas of Agency and 'Choice' for Feminism: A Reply to Duits and van Zoonen." *European Journal of Women's Studies* 14 (1): 69–80.

———. 2007b. "Postfeminist Media Culture: Elements of a Sensibility." *European Journal of Cultural Studies* 10 (2): 147–166.

Gillespie, Rosemary. 1996. "Women, the Body and Brand Extension in Medicine: Cosmetic Surgery and the Paradox of Choice." *Women and Health* 24 (4): 69–85.

Gilman, Sander L. 1999. *Making the Body Beautiful: A Cultural History of Aesthetic Surgery*. Princeton, NJ: Princeton University Press.

Gimlin, Debra. 2000. "Cosmetic Surgery: Beauty as Commodity." *Qualitative Sociology* 23 (1): 77–98.

———. 2007. "Accounting for Cosmetic Surgery in the USA and Great Britain: A Cross-cultural Analysis of Women's Narratives." *Body and Society* 13 (1): 41–60.

———. 2010. "Imagining the Other in Cosmetic Surgery." *Body and Society* 16 (4): 57–76.

———. 2012. *Cosmetic Surgery Narratives: A Cross-Cultural Analysis of Women's Accounts*. New York: Palgrave Macmillan.

———. 2013. "'Too Good to Be Real': The Obviously Augmented Breast in Women's Narratives of Cosmetic Surgery." *Gender and Society* 27 (6): 913–934.

Goffman, Erving. 1959. *The Presentation of Self in Everyday Life*. Garden City, NY: Doubleday.

———. 1963. *Stigma: Notes on the Management of Spoiled Identity*. Englewood Cliffs, NJ: Prentice-Hall.

Gravelin, Claire R., Monica Biernat, and Matthew Baldwin. 2017. "The Impact of Power and Powerlessness on Blaming the Victim of Sexual Assault." *Group Processes and Intergroup Relations* 22 (1): 98–115.

Gravelin, Claire R., Monica Biernat, and Caroline E. Bucher. 2018. "Blaming the Victim of Acquaintance Rape: Individual, Situational, and Sociocultural Factors." *Frontiers in Psychology* 9:2422.

Haiken, Elizabeth. 1997. *Venus Envy: A History of Cosmetic Surgery*. Baltimore, MD: Johns Hopkins University Press.

Hakim, Catherine. 2010. "Erotic Capital." *European Sociological Review* 26 (5): 499–518.

Hamermesh, Daniel S. 2011. *Beauty Pays: Why Attractive People Are More Successful*. Princeton, NJ: Princeton University Press.

Hanbury, Mary. 2018. "These Photos Reveal Why Women Are Abandoning Victoria's Secret for American Eagle's Aerie Underwear Brand." *Business Insider*, July 20. Available at http://www.businessinsider.com/women-abandon-victorias-secret-for-aerie-photos-2018-2.

Hays, Sharon. 1994. "Structure and Agency and the Sticky Problem of Culture." *Sociological Theory* 12 (1): 57–72.

Heyes, Cressida J., and Meredith Jones, eds. 2009. *Cosmetic Surgery: A Feminist Primer*. Burlington, VT: Ashgate.

Hill, Catherine, and Holly Kearl. 2011. *Crossing the Line: Sexual Harassment at School*. Washington, DC: American Association of University Women.

Hoffman, Nathan. 2015. "Achieve the Final Results Patients Desire." *Dental Lab Products* 40 (9): 12–14.

Honigman, Roberta J., Katharine A. Phillips, and David J. Castle. 2004. "A Review of Psychosocial Outcomes for Patients Seeking Cosmetic Surgery." *Plastic and Reconstructive Surgery* 113 (4): 1129–1237.

hooks, bell. 2000. *Where We Stand: Class Matters*. New York: Routledge.

Howard, Jacqueline, and Anna Ginsburg. 2018. "The History of the 'Ideal' Woman and Where That Has Left Us." *CNN*, March 9. Available at: https://www.cnn.com/2018/03/07/health/body-image-history-of-beauty-explainer-intl/index.html.

Huis in 't Veld, Eva A., Francisco L. Canales, and Heather J. Furnas. 2017. "The Impact of a Plastic Surgeon's Gender on Patient Choice." *Aesthetic Surgery Journal* 37 (4): 466–471.

Hunter, Margaret L. 2002. "'If You're Light You're Alright': Light Skin Color as Social Capital for Women of Color." *Gender and Society* 16 (2): 175–193.

———. 2005. *Race, Gender, and the Politics of Skin Tone*. New York: Routledge.

———. 2011. "Buying Racial Capital: Skin-Bleaching and Cosmetic Surgery in a Globalized World." *Journal of Pan African Studies* 4 (4): 142–164.

Ishigooka, Jun, Mitsuhiro Iwao, Makihiko Suzuki, Yoshitsuna Fukuyama, Mitsukuni Muraska, and Sadanori Miura. 1998. "Demographic Features of Patients Seeking Cosmetic Surgery." *Psychiatry and Clinical Neurosciences* 52 (3): 283–287.

Jamaluddin, Lira. 2015. "21 Quotes from Madonna," *Marie Claire*, August 17. Available at http://marieclaire.com.my/latest-news/21-quotes-from-madonna/.

Janzen, Sydney. 2015. "Amending Rape Shield Laws: Outdated Statutes Fail to Protect Victims on Social Media." *John Marshall Law Review* 48 (4): 1087–1118.

Jeffreys, Sheila. 2015. *Beauty and Misogyny: Harmful Cultural Practices in the West*. 2nd ed. New York: Routledge.

Jha, Meeta Rani. 2016. *The Global Beauty Industry: Colorism, Racism, and the National Body*. New York: Routledge.

Johns Hopkins Medicine. n.d. "Types of Surgery." Available at https://www.hopkinsmedicine.org/healthlibrary/conditions/surgical_care/types_of_surgery_85,P01416 (accessed December 11, 2019).

Jones, Meredith. 2008. *Skintight: An Anatomy of Cosmetic Surgery*. New York: Berg.

Kaiser, Susan B., Carla M. Freeman, and Stacy B. Wingate. 1985. "Stigmata and Negotiated Outcomes: Management of Appearance by Persons with Physical Disabilities." *Deviant Behavior* 6 (2): 205–224.

Kang, Milliann. 2010. *The Managed Hand: Race, Gender, and the Body in Beauty Service Work*. Berkeley: University of California Press.

Kates, Steven M., and Glenda Shaw-Garlock. 1999. "The Ever Entangling Web: A Study of Ideologies and Discourses in Advertising to Women." *Journal of Advertising* 28 (2): 33–49.

Kaw, Eugenia. 1993. "Medicalization of Racial Features: Asian American Women and Cosmetic Surgery." *Medical Anthropology Quarterly* 7 (1): 74–89.

"Kendall Jenner Height Weight, Waist, Hip Measurement." 2015. *Heightline*, November 7. Available at https://heightline.com/kendall-jenner-height-weight-waist-hip-measurement/.

Kim, David C., Soo Kim, and Amit Mitra. 1997. "Perceptions and Misconceptions of the Plastic and Reconstructive Surgeon." *Annals of Plastic Surgery* 38 (4): 426–430.

Kim, Janna L., C. Lynn Sorsoli, Katherine Collins, Bonnie A. Zylbergold, Deborah Schooler, and Deborah L. Tolman. 2007. "From Sex to Sexuality: Exposing the Heterosexual Script on Primetime Network Television." *Journal of Sex Research* 44 (2): 145–157.

King, Nina-Marie H., Vedran R. Lovric, William C. R. Parr, W. R. Walsh, and Pourla R. Moradi. 2017. "What Is the Standard Volume to Increase a Cup Size for Breast Augmentation Surgery? A Novel Three-Dimensional Computer Tomographic Approach." *Plastic and Reconstructive Surgery* 139 (5): 1084–1089.

Kvaale, Erlend P., Nick Haslam, and William H. Gottdiener. 2013. "The 'Side Effects' of Medicalization: A Meta-analytic Review of How Biogenetic Explanations Affect Stigma." *Clinical Psychology Review* 33 (6): 782–794.

Kwan, Samantha. 2010. "Navigating Public Spaces: Gender, Race, and Body Privilege in Everyday Life." *Feminist Formations* 22 (2): 144–166.

Kwan, Samantha, and Jennifer Graves. 2013. *Framing Fat: Competing Constructions in Contemporary Culture*. New Brunswick, NJ: Rutgers University Press.

Kwan, Samantha, and Mary Nell Trautner. 2009. "Beauty Work: Individual and Institutional Rewards, the Reproduction of Gender, and Questions of Agency." *Sociology Compass* 3 (1): 49–71.

Lamont, Michèle. 1992. *Money, Morals, and Manners: The Culture of the French and American Upper-Middle Class*. Chicago: University of Chicago Press.

Lamont, Michèle, and Virág Molnár. 2002. "The Study of Boundaries in the Social Sciences." *Annual Review of Sociology* 28:167–195.

Lamont, Michèle, Sabrina Pendergrass, and Mark C. Pachucki. 2015. "Symbolic Boundaries." In *International Encyclopedia of the Social and Behavioral Sciences*, vol. 23, 2nd ed., edited by James Wright, 850–855. New York: Elsevier.

Lawton, Tenley. 2018. "Will You Need To Replace Your Breast Implants?" American Society of Plastic Surgeons. January 23. Available at https://

www.plasticsurgery.org/news/blog/will-you-need-to-replace-your-breast
-implants.

Leeds, Maxine. 1994. "Young African-American Women and the Language of Beauty." In *Ideals of Feminine Beauty: Philosophical, Social, and Cultural Dimensions*, edited by Karen A. Callaghan, 147–160. Westport, CT: Greenwood Press.

Lehrman, Karen. 1997. *The Lipstick Proviso: Women, Sex and Power in the Real World*. New York: Doubleday.

Li, Shan. 2016. "Barbie Breaks the Mold with Ethnically Diverse Dolls." *Los Angeles Times*, January 28. Available at https://www.latimes.com/business/la-fi-mattel-barbie-20160128-story.html.

Linton, Simi. 1998. *Claiming Disability: Knowledge and Disability*. New York: New York University Press.

L'Oréal. n.d. "Dermablend." Available at http://www.lorealusa.com/brand/active-cosmetics-division/dermablend (accessed December 11, 2019).

Lukács, Georg. (1923) 1971. *History and Class Consciousness: Studies in Marxist Dialectics*. Translated by Rodney Livingstone. Cambridge, MA: MIT Press.

Mann, Traci, A. Janet Tomiyama, Erika Westling, Ann-Marie Lew, Barbra Samuels, and Jason Chatman. 2007. "Medicare's Search for Effective Obesity Treatments: Diets Are Not the Answer." *American Psychologist* 62 (3): 220–233.

Markey, Charlotte N., and Patrick M. Markey. 2015. "Can Women's Body Image Be 'Fixed'? Women's Bodies, Well-Being, and Cosmetic Surgery." In *The Wrong Prescription for Women: How Medicine and Media Create a "Need" for Treatments, Drugs, and Surgery*, edited by Maureen C. McHugh and Joan C. Chrisler, 221–237. Santa Barbara, CA: Praeger.

Mason, Katherine. 2012. "The Unequal Weight of Discrimination: Gender, Body Size, and Income Inequality." *Social Problems* 59 (3): 411–435.

Mayo Clinic. 2017. "Cosmetic Surgery." July 19. Available at https://www.mayoclinic.org/tests-procedures/cosmetic-surgery/about/pac-20385138.

———. 2018. "MRSA Infection." October 18. Available at https://www.mayoclinic.org/diseases-conditions/mrsa/symptoms-causes/syc-20375336.

McGee, Micki. 2005. *Self-Help, Inc.: Makeover Culture in American Life*. New York: Oxford University Press.

McHugh, Maureen, and Joan C. Chrisler. 2015. "Introduction: The Medicalization of Women's Bodies and Everyday Experiences." In *The Wrong Prescription for Women: How Medicine and Media Create a "Need" for Treatments, Drugs, and Surgery*, edited by Maureen C. McHugh, and Joan C. Chrisler, 1–16. Santa Barbara, CA: Praeger.

McRobbie, Angela. 2009. *The Aftermath of Feminism: Gender, Culture and Social Change*. Los Angeles: SAGE.

Mead, George Herbert. 1934. *Mind, Self, and Society*. Chicago: University of Chicago Press.

Minsberg, Talya. 2018. "Runners Practiced in Sports Bras; Rowan University Told Them to Go Elsewhere." *New York Times*, November 9. Available at https://www.nytimes.com/2018/11/09/sports/rowan-sports-bra-controversy .html.

Molloy, Beth L., and Sharon D. Herzberger. 1998. "Body Image and Self-Esteem: A Comparison of African-American and Caucasian Women." *Sex Roles* 38 (7–8): 631–643.

Morgan, Kathryn Pauly. 1991. "Women and the Knife: Cosmetic Surgery and Colonization of Women's Bodies." *Hypatia* 6 (3): 25–53.

Motakef, Saba, Sahar Motakef, Michael T. Chung, Michael J. Ingargiola, and Jose Rodriguez-Feliz. 2014. "The Cosmetic Surgery Stigma: An American Cultural Phenomenon?" *Plastic and Reconstructive Surgery* 134 (5): 854e–855e.

Mull, Amanda. 2019. "America Is Too Glib about Breast Implants." *The Atlantic*, March 27. Available at https://www.theatlantic.com/health/archive/2019/ 03/fda-breast-implants/585829/?fbclid=IwAR37EGl5m9In8WIDYQ4Z5x -WgsRvIXFd-lsykUPdzAE5kh9Vclddyu5mmVg.

Mulvey, Laura. 1989. *Visual and Other Pleasures*. Bloomington, IN: Indianapolis University Press.

Nash, Meredith, and Ruby Grant. 2015. "Twenty-Something *Girls* v. Thirty-Something *Sex and the City* Women: Paving the Way for 'Post? Feminism.'" *Feminist Media Studies* 15 (6): 976–991.

National Organization for Women. n.d. "About." Available at https://now.org/ now-foundation/love-your-body/love-your-body-whats-it-all-about/about/ (accessed December 11, 2019).

Naugler, Diane. 2010. "'Oh, Sure They're Nice, but Are They Real?' Greeting Cards and the Normalizing of Cosmetic Surgical Intervention in Practices of Feminine Embodiment." *Resources for Feminist Research* 33 (3–4): 119–135.

Negra, Diane. 2009. *What a Girl Wants? Fantasizing the Reclamation of Self in Postfeminism*. New York: Routledge.

Norton, Kevin I., Timothy S. Olds, Scott Olive, and Stephen Dank. 1996. "Ken and Barbie at Life Size." *Sex Roles* 34 (3–4): 287–294.

Omi, Michael, and Howard Winant. 1994. *Racial Formation in the United States: From the 1960s to the 1990s*. 2nd ed. New York: Routledge.

Paquette, Marie-Claude, and Kim Raine. 2004. "Sociocultural Context of Women's Body Image." *Social Science and Medicine* 59 (5): 1047–1058.

Park, Kristin. 2002. "Stigma Management among the Voluntarily Childless." *Sociological Perspectives* 45 (1): 21–45.

Parker, Sheila, Mimi Nichter, Mark Nichter, Nancy Vuckovic, Colette Sims, and Cheryl Ritenbaugh. 1995. "Body Image and Weight Concerns among African American and White Adolescent Females: Differences That Make a Difference." *Human Organization* 54 (2): 103–114.

Parsons, Talcott. 1951. *The Social System.* Glencoe, IL: Free Press.

Paxton, Susan J., Dianne Neumark-Sztainer, Peter J. Hannon, and Marla E. Eisenberg. 2006. "Body Dissatisfaction Prospectively Predicts Depressed Mood and Low Self-Esteem in Girls and Boys." *Journal of Clinical Child and Adolescent Psychology* 35 (4): 539–549.

Petersen, William. 1966. "Success Story, Japanese-American Style." *New York Times Magazine,* January 9. Available at https://www.nytimes.com/1966/01/09/archives/success-story-japaneseamerican-style-success-story-japaneseamerican.html.

Pew Research Center. 2018. "The Data on Women Leaders." September 13. Available at http://www.pewsocialtrends.org/fact-sheet/the-data-on-women-leaders/.

Pitts-Taylor, Victoria. 2007. *Surgery Junkies: Wellness and Pathology in Cosmetic Culture.* New Brunswick, NJ: Rutgers University Press.

———. 2009. "Becoming/Being a Cosmetic Surgery Patient: Semantic Instability and the Intersubjective Self." *Studies in Gender and Sexuality* 10 (3): 119–128.

Prendergast, Tahira I., Sharon K. Ong'uti, Gezzer Ortega, Amal L. Khoury, Ekene Onwuka, Oluwaseyi B. Bolorunduro, Edward E. Cornwell III, and Henry Paul Jr. 2011. "Differential Trends in Racial Preferences for Cosmetic Procedures." *American Surgeon* 77 (8): 1081–1085.

Puhl, Rebecca M., and Chelsea A. Heuer. 2009. "The Stigma of Obesity: A Review and Update." *Obesity* 17 (5): 941–964.

Ray, Ranita. 2018. "Identity of Distance: How Economically Marginalized Black and Latina Women Navigate Risk Discourse and Employ Feminist Ideals." *Social Problems* 65 (4): 456–472.

Rhode, Deborah L. 2010. *The Beauty Bias: The Injustice of Appearance in Life and Law.* New York: Oxford University Press.

Riessman, Catherine K. 1983. "Women and Medicalization: A New Perspective." *Social Policy* 14 (1): 3–18.

Robehmed, Natalie. 2018. "Highest-Paid Models 2018: Kendall Jenner Leads with $22.5 Million." *Forbes,* December 13. Available at https://www.forbes.com/sites/natalierobehmed/2018/12/13/highest-paid-models-2018-kendall-jenner-leads-with-22-5-million/#61499e443ddf.

Rodin, Judith, Lisa Silberstein, and Ruth Striegel-Moore. 1984. "Women and Weight: A Normative Discontent." *Nebraska Symposium on Motivation* 32:267–307.

Roman, Denise. 2011. "Under the Rape Shield: Constitutional and Feminist Critiques of Rape Shield Laws." *CSW Update,* April 4. Available at https://escholarship.org/uc/item/31t8d960.

Ronai, Carol Rambo. 1994. "Narrative Resistance to Deviance: Identity Management among Strip-Tease Dancers." *Perspectives on Social Problems* 6:195–213.

Runfola, Cristin D., Ann Von Holle, Sara E. Trace, Kimberly A. Brownley, Sara M. Hofmeier, Danielle A. Gagne, and Cynthia M. Bulik. 2013. "Body Dissatisfaction in Women across the Lifespan: Results of the UNC-*SELF* and Gender and Body Image (GABI) Studies." *European Eating Disorders Review* 21 (1): 52–59.

Sanchez Taylor, Jacqueline. 2012. "Fake Breasts and Power: Gender, Class and Cosmetic Surgery." *Women's Studies International Forum* 35 (6): 458–466.

Sansone, Randy A., and Lori A. Sansone. 2007. "Cosmetic Surgery and Psychological Issues." *Psychiatry* 4 (12): 65–68.

Sarwer, David B., Lauren M. Gibbons, Leanne Magee, James L. Baker, Laurie A. Casas, Paul M. Glat, Alan H. Gold, Mark L. Jewell, Don LaRossa, Foad Nahai, and V. Leroy Young. 2005. "A Prospective, Multi-site Investigation of Patient Satisfaction and Psychosocial Status following Cosmetic Surgery." *Aesthetic Surgery Journal* 25 (3): 263–269.

Saxena, Preeta. 2013. "Trading and Managing Stigma: Women's Accounts of Breast Implant Surgery." *Journal of Contemporary Ethnography* 42 (3): 347–377.

Scott, Marvin B., and Stanford M. Lyman. 1968. "Accounts." *American Sociological Review* 33 (1): 46–62.

Seattle Plastic Surgery. 2013. "Breaking Down the Stereotypes about Plastic Surgeons." August 30. Available at http://www.seattleplasticsurgery.com/2013/08/breaking-down-the-stereotypes-about-plastic-surgeons/.

Shannon, Joel. 2018. "Plastic Surgeon 'Dr. Bumbum' Arrested in Brazil after Patient Dies following Butt Enhancement Surgery." *USA Today*, July 20. Available at https://www.usatoday.com/story/news/world/2018/07/20/dr-bumbum-arrested-brazil-after-patient-dies/805209002.

Shilling, Chris. 2012. *The Body and Social Theory.* 3rd ed. Los Angeles: SAGE.

Siegel, Karolynn, Howard Lune, and Ilan H. Meyer. 1998. "Stigma Management among Gay/Bisexual Men with HIV/AIDS." *Qualitative Sociology* 21 (1): 3–24.

Silva, Amanda K., Aviva Preminger, Sheri Slezak, Linda G. Phillips, and Debra J. Johnson. 2016. "Melting the Plastic Ceiling: Overcoming Obstacles to Foster Leadership in Women Plastic Surgeons." *Plastic and Reconstructive Surgery* 138 (3): 721–729.

Simon, William, and John H. Gagnon. 1986. "Sexual Scripts: Permanence and Change." *Archives of Sexual Behavior* 15 (2): 97–120.

Sischo, Lacey, and Patricia Yancey Martin. 2015. "The Price of Femininity or Just Pleasing Myself? Justifying Breast Surgery." *Gender Issues* 32 (2): 77–96.

Smith, Sharon G., Xinjian Zhang, Kathleen C. Basile, Melissa T. Merrick, Jing Wang, Marci-Jo Kresnow, and Jieru Chen. 2018. "The National Intimate Partner and Sexual Violence Survey: 2015 Data Brief—Updated Release." Available at https://www.cdc.gov/violenceprevention/pdf/2015data-brief508.pdf.

Snow, David A., and Leon Anderson. 1987. "Identity Work among the Homeless: The Verbal Construction and Avowal of Personal Identities." *American Journal of Sociology* 92 (6): 1336–1371.

Stafford, Barbara M., John La Puma, and David L. Schiedermayer. 1989. "One Face of Beauty, One Picture of Health: The Hidden Aesthetic of Medical Practice." *Journal of Medicine and Philosophy* 14 (2): 213–230.

Stanley, Jessamyn. 2017. *Let Go of Fear, Get on the Mat, Love Your Body*. New York: Workman.

Stuart, Avelie, Tim Kurz, and Kerry Ashby. 2012. "Damned If You and Damned If You Don't': The (Re)Production of Larger Breasts as Ideal in Criticisms of Breast Surgery." *Australian Feminist Studies* 27 (74): 405–420.

Sudnow, David. 1967. *Passing On: The Social Organization of Dying*. Englewood Cliffs, NJ: Prentice-Hall.

Sullivan, Deborah A. 2001. *Cosmetic Surgery: The Cutting Edge of Commercial Medicine in America*. New Brunswick, NJ: Rutgers University Press.

Swami, Viren, Angela Nogueira Campana, and Rebecca Coles. 2012. "Acceptance of Cosmetic Surgery among British Female University Students: Are There Ethnic Differences?" *European Psychologist* 17 (1): 55–62.

Sykes, Gresham M., and David Matza. 1957. "Techniques of Neutralization: A Theory of Delinquency." *American Sociological Review* 22 (6): 664–670.

Tait, Sue. 2007. "Television and the Domestication of Cosmetic Surgery." *Feminist Media Studies* 7 (2): 119–135.

"'The Talk' Ladies Host Show without Makeup." 2012. *Huffington Post*, September 10. Available at https://www.huffingtonpost.com/2012/09/10/the-talk-no-makeup_n_1872001.html.

Talley, Heather Laine. 2014. *Saving Face: Disfigurement and the Politics of Appearance*. New York: New York University Press.

Tam, Kim-Pong, Henry Kin-Shing Ng, Young-Hoon Kim, Victoria Wai-Lan Yeung, and Francis Yue-Lok Cheung. 2012. "Attitudes toward Cosmetic Surgery Patients: The Role of Culture and Social Contact." *Journal of Social Psychology* 152 (4): 458–579.

Tanenbaum, Leora. 2015. *I Am Not a Slut: Slut-Shaming in the Age of the Internet*. New York: Harper Perennial.

Tanna, Neil, Nitin J. Patel, Hamdan Azhar, and Jay W. Granzow. 2010. "Professional Perceptions of Plastic and Reconstructive Surgery: What Primary Care Physicians Think." *Plastic and Reconstructive Surgery* 126 (2): 643–650.

Tanne, Janice Hopkins. 2003. "New US Drama Outrages Plastic Surgeons." *British Medical Journal* 327 (7409): 295.

Thompson, Craig J., and Diane L. Haytko. 1997. "Speaking of Fashion: Consumers' Uses of Fashion Discourses and the Appropriation of Countervailing Cultural Meanings." *Journal of Consumer Research* 24 (1): 15–42.

Throsby, Karen. 2008. "Happy Re-birthday: Weight Loss Surgery and the 'New Me.'" *Body and Society* 14 (1): 117–133.

Timmermans, Stefan. 1998. "Social Death as a Self-Fulfilling Prophecy: David Sudnow's *Passing On* Revisited." *Sociological Quarterly* 39 (3): 453–472.

Toerien, Merran, Sue Wilkinson, and Precilla Y. L. Choi. 2005. "Body Hair Removal: The 'Mundane' Production of Normative Femininity." *Sex Roles* 52 (5–6): 399–406.

Turner, Jacob S. 2011. "Sex and the Spectacle of Music Videos: An Examination of the Portrayal of Race and Sexuality in Music Videos." *Sex Roles* 64 (3–4): 173–191.

U.S. Census Bureau. 2018. "Sex by Age." Available at https://censusreporter.org/data/table/?table=B01001&primary_geo_id=01000US&geo_ids=01000US.

U.S. Department of Health and Human Services. 2017. "2017 Poverty Guidelines." Available at https://aspe.hhs.gov/2017-poverty-guidelines.

U.S. Food and Drug Administration. 2011. "FDA Update on the Safety of Silicone Gel–Filled Breast Implants." June. Available at https://www.fda.gov/downloads/MedicalDevices/ProductsandMedicalProcedures/ImplantsandProsthetics/BreastImplants/UCM260090.pdf.

———. 2018. "Photographs and/or Illustrations of Breast Implant Complications." January 18. Available at https://www.fda.gov/medical-devices/breast-implants/photographs-andor-illustrations-breast-implant-complications.

———. 2019. "Risks and Complications of Breast Implants." Available at https://www.fda.gov/medical-devices/breast-implants/risks-and-complications-breast-implants.

Vannini, Phillip, and Aaron M. McCright. 2004. "To Die For: The Semiotic Seductive Power of the Tanned Body." *Symbolic Interaction* 27 (3): 309–332.

Veblen, Thorstein. (1899) 1994. *The Theory of the Leisure Class.* New York: Dover.

Verner, Amy. 2011. "L'Oréal's 'Because I'm Worth It' Slogan Marks a Milestone." *Globe and Mail*, December 2. Available at https://www.theglobeandmail.com/life/fashion-and-beauty/beauty/loreals-because-im-worth-it-slogan-marks-a-milestone/article554604/.

Weber, Brenda R. 2009. *Makeover TV: Selfhood, Citizenship, and Celebrity.* Durham, NC: Duke University Press.

WebMD. 2019a. "Breast Implants." July 25. Available at https://www.webmd.com/beauty/cosmetic-procedures-breast-augmentation#1.

———. 2019b. "Breast Implant Safety." February 3. Available at https://www.webmd.com/beauty/breast-implant-safety#.

———. 2019c. "Cosmetic Procedures: Scars." August 27. Available at https://www.webmd.com/beauty/cosmetic-procedures-scars#1.

Webster, Murray, Jr., and James E. Driskell Jr. 1983. "Beauty as Status." *American Journal of Sociology* 89 (1): 140–165.

Weisman, Aly. 2012. "Breaking Breakdown: How Jennifer Aniston Spends $141,037 on Her Red Carpet Regimen." *Business Insider*, March 8. Available at https://www.businessinsider.com/beauty-breakdown-how-jennifer-aniston-spends-141037-on-her-red-carpet-regimen-2012-3.

Weitz, Rose. 2001. "Women and Their Hair: Seek Power through Resistance and Accommodation." *Gender and Society* 15 (5): 667–686.

West, Candace, and Don H. Zimmerman. 1987. "Doing Gender." *Gender and Society* 1 (2): 125–151.

Whelehan, Imelda. 2010. "Remaking Feminism: Or Why Is Postfeminism So Boring?" *Nordic Journal of English Studies* 9 (3): 155–172.

Wolf, Naomi. 1992. *The Beauty Myth: How Images of Beauty Are Used Against Women.* New York: Anchor Books.

———. 1997. *Promiscuities: The Secret Struggle for Womanhood.* New York: Random House.

Young, Cathy. 1993. "The New Madonna/Whore Syndrome: Feminism, Sexuality, and Sexual Harassment." *New York Law School Law Review* 38:257–288.

Young, Iris Marion. 1992. "Breasted Experience: The Look and the Feeling." In *The Body in Medical Thought and Practice*, edited by Drew Leder, 215–230. Boston: Kluwer.

Index

Samantha Kwan is an Associate Professor of Sociology at the University of Houston. Her research focuses on how people embody, resist, and negotiate body norms and scripts. She is coauthor of *Framing Fat: Competing Constructions in Contemporary Culture* and coeditor of *Embodied Resistance: Challenging the Norms, Breaking the Rules; The Politics of Women's Bodies: Sexuality, Appearance, and Behavior*; and *Body Battlegrounds: Transgressions, Tensions, and Transformations.*

Jennifer Graves is a Lecturer of Sociology at the University of Houston. Her research focuses on the sociology of the body and embodiment with a particular interest in fat studies. She is coauthor of *Framing Fat: Competing Constructions in Contemporary Culture.*

Printed by Printforce, United Kingdom